MANIFEST A LIFE
WITH CLARITY, CAL

365 DAYS OF MORNING MAGIC

A DAILY GUIDE TO SET YOUR INTENTIONS

Emma Walkinshaw

Introduction

This little book you're holding found its spark in the afterglow of a 6 am yoga class at my cozy studio on Chevron Island, Gold Coast, Australia. Picture this: as I strolled to my car, the magic of a morning practice lingered, like a gift that just keeps giving all day long.

In that moment, a realization washed over me. - not everyone gets to dive into their day like this. Life, with its demands like parenthood and work, often nudges us away from these peaceful mornings. So, here's my thought: what if we distilled it down to three simple steps, each just 7 minutes long? Seven minutes of yoga, another seven for meditation or a mantra, and a sweet seven for flowetry – like journaling, but with your pen dancing freely on paper in a blissful flow state.

I get it; keeping up a morning ritual is tough without some accountability. These three steps? Consider them your friendly guide to a soulful morning practice.

My wish for you? Move your beautiful body with ease and grace, let a positive mantra nestle in your heart and mind, and when you put pen to paper, let those flowetry prompts take your mind on a joyful journey. It's not just a moment for reflection; it's shaping a purposeful day, week, or year. May your heart dance with passion, your mind stay sharp, and your body flow with ease and grace.

The power of 21 minutes may sound simple, but trust me, it's pure magic. You deserve these moments to sit with yourself, to tune into your inner wisdom.

So, today, let's listen to that intuition. Today, let's be true to ourselves and, in turn, to others. And above all, today, let's infuse everything we do with love and compassion, starting with ourselves and rippling out to the world.

Namaste,
Emma

DISCLAIMER: PLEASE READ CAREFULLY

The 365 days of Morning Magic Book is not a substitute for coaching or therapy. It provides educational and inspirational content for personal growth. By participating, you acknowledge:

- Not a Replacement: This book is not a substitute for professional coaching or therapy.

- Personal Responsibility: You are responsible for your well-being and should adapt practices to your needs.

- No Guarantee: This book does not guarantee specific results or outcomes.

- Consultation: If you have health concerns, consult with professionals before starting

Dedication

To my beloved Brendon,
Thank you for being you. Your unshakable love and support, your tolerance, your ease and kindness, your strength your tenderness and allowance for me to show up as I am and you love me in all my many versions and stages of Emma. You have my heart and soul.

Ruby & Sonny- You are my greatest achievements. I love you both more than any words could ever express.

Acknowledgment

I would like to express my deepest gratitude to my family for their unwavering support and encouragement. To my parents, Marg and Jack, thank you for always believing in me. To my beloved husband, Brendon, and my children, Ruby and Sonny, your love means the world to me. I'd also like to thank my Nana Ursula, who made me the woman I am today. You showed me how to connect with others with warmth, compassion, and a little bit of cheekiness. And I'd also like to thank my mother-in-law, Niecy. I love you all more than words can express. I consider myself the richest woman alive because I have you all.

I would also like to acknowledge my friends who contributed and helped me stay accountable and on track. Kim, you have kept me sane, always being honest, giving helpful feedback, and making me laugh until my belly hurts and tears run down my cheeks.

Acknowledgment

Thank you, Belsy (Belinda White), for the front cover and design of the book. Your creativity, kindness, and generosity of time and energy are greatly appreciated.

To all the women who have joined me in Clarity Catalyst, Yoga in Paradise, Embody Me Program, Wholehearted Retreats, and my thriving 21 Minutes of Morning Magic community, and all the workshops and events, thank you for saying YES. Each and every one of you is an inspiration and the reason why I do what I do.

Thank you all for being a part of this journey.

Namaste,
Em xx

Testimonials

This morning practice really sets the tone of my day and I notice the different on the days I don't do it. It helps me be a lot more present during the day.
~Jane~

I think it is the most beautiful
gift you can give yourself.
~Kirsti~

The most significant impact 21 MMM had in my life is Regular spiritual practice, Inward focus, Peace, Deeper sense of myself and Soul connection.
~Emily~

I have been guided into beautiful meditations and now I am calmer and able to start the day with clarity. I also gained so much more self awareness with the journaling.
~Gini~

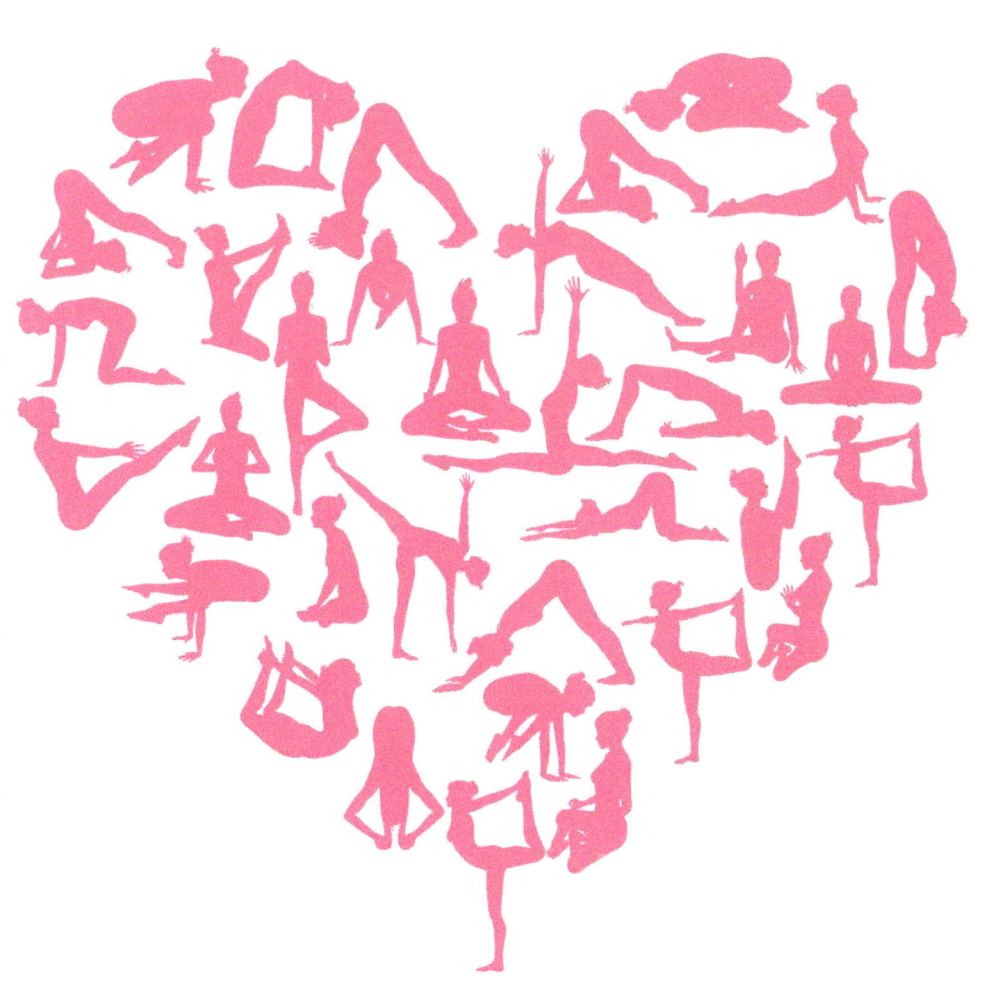

Create your Morning Magic Space

Prepare your sacred morning space by laying out a yoga mat, a cozy cushion, and gather your tools - a pen, journal, and a refreshing sip of water. Open your heart and mind to the transformative power of flowetry, a simple yet profound practice of letting creative words gently spill onto the page. Approach this 21-minute ritual with no expectations, allowing your inner creativity to blossom. This intentional morning magic will leave you grounded, inspired, and connected to the essence of your soul.

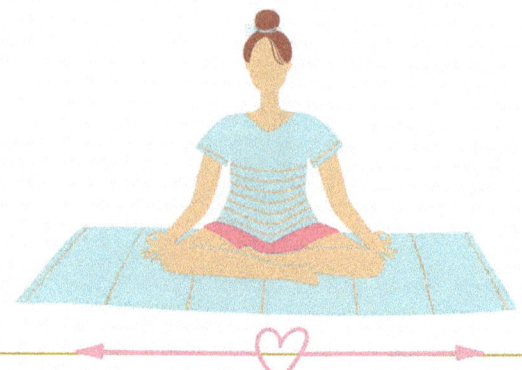

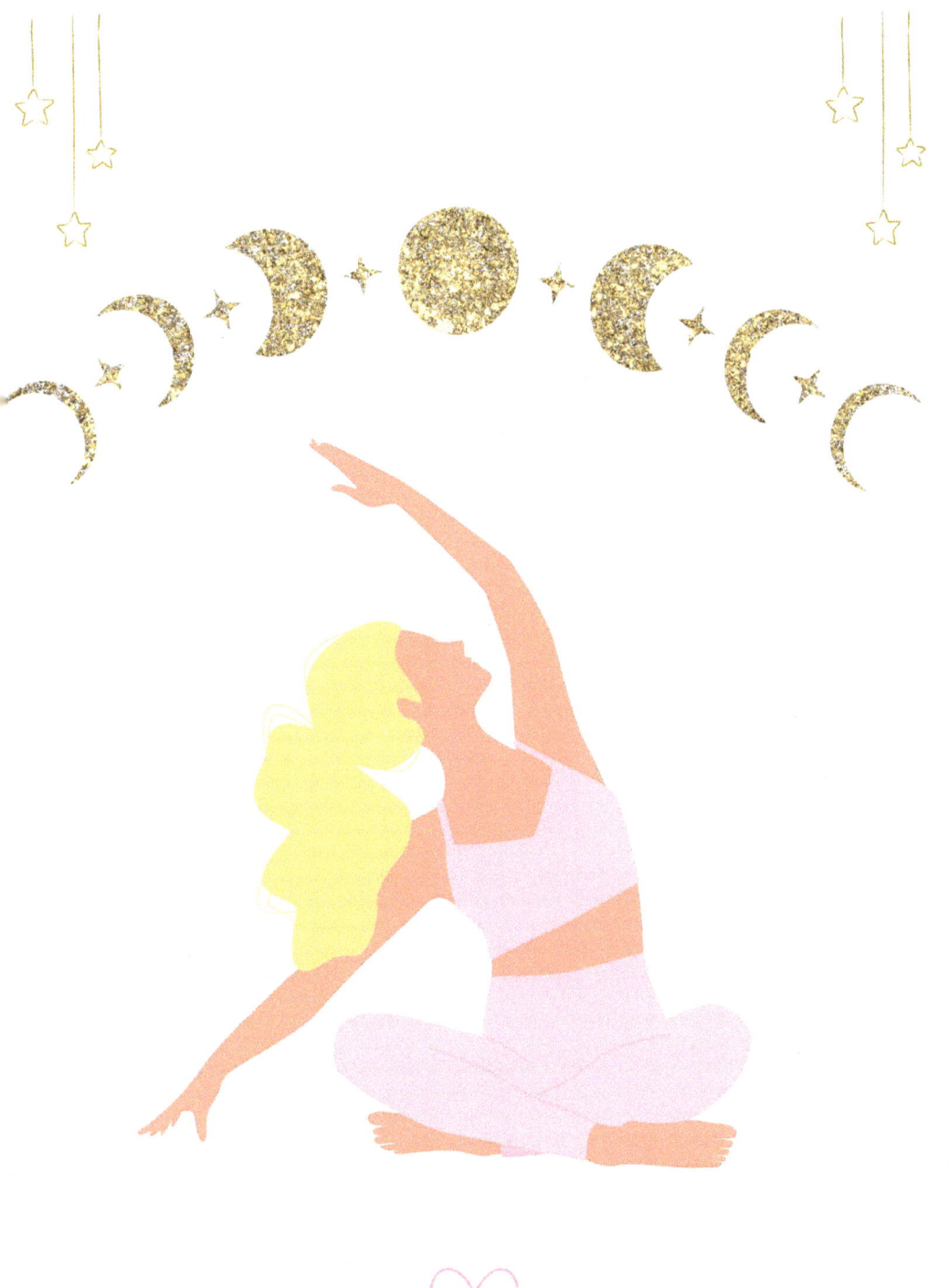

January

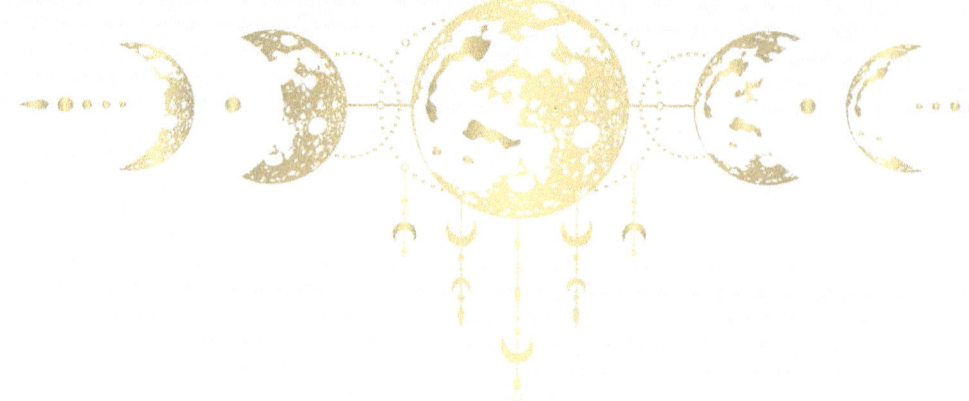

My heart's desire

Happy New year and blessings to an abundant year ahead! Let's Embrace the magic of a new year, be fearless, and chase your dreams. Let's create a year full of adventure, joy, and courage. Open your heart, let love flow like never before. You've got another lap around the sun. Dream big, live boldly, and cherish every heartbeat. Embrace the sacred rhythm of 21 minutes in your morning magic practice. With the gentle flow of yoga, the stillness of meditation, and the soulful expression of flowetry, you're opening the doors to a realm where clarity and inspiration dance hand in hand. As you honor this ritual, watch how the universe responds, bestowing upon you a deeper connection and a wellspring of inner light that grows with each devoted moment.

January 1st

New Energy

Embracing the new energy of the year. Opening to new possibilities. Thanking last year and welcoming the new year.

Meditation & Mantra

I live in a prosperous world.

Flowetry Prompts

What has mother nature taught me about prosperity?

January 2nd

Fresh Start

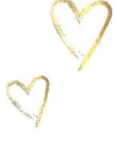 Clean up, clean out, give away, pass onto someone else. Declutter your space. Let's welcome fresh energy.

Meditation & Mantra

I am energy.

Flowetry Prompts

What do I need to declutter in my life?

January 3rd

Make Real

The meaning of Manifest is to "Make Real" through inspired actions & beliefs.

Meditation & Mantra

I create a life I love.

Flowetry Prompts

What am I going to "Make Real" this year?

January 4th

Manifestation of the heart

This year, I set my intention, focusing on my deepest heart's desire, defining what I want, how I want to feel, and listening to my heart's true longing.

Meditation & Mantra

I listen to my heart's desire.

Flowetry Prompts

Setting my intention for this year. What does my heart want to manifest?

January 5th

Spirituality and Inner Growth

Set intentions for personal growth, spiritual connection, self-discovery, and the exploration of your spiritual path.

Meditation & Mantra
This year I focus on inner growth.

Flowetry Prompts
Setting my intentions for this year's personal/spiritual growth.

January 6th

Adventure and Exploration

Embrace the adventurous spirit within you. Set intentions for exploring new horizons, whether through travel, learning, or embarking on new experiences that enrich your life.

Meditation & Mantra

I live an enriched life.

Flowetry Prompts

Setting my intentions for this year. Where and what do I want to explore & experience?

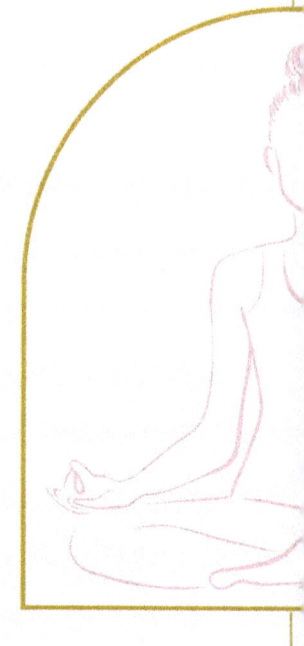

January 7th

Inner and Outer Radiance

Prioritize self-love, self-compassion, and physical and emotional well-being. Set intentions for maintaining a healthy lifestyle, practicing mindfulness, and nurturing your body and mind.

Meditation & Mantra

Radiance is my essence.

Flowetry Prompts

What's one thing I want to change or improve in my life this year? How can I make it happen?

January 8th

Nature Connection

Make an effort to connect with nature, being fully present and immersed in the outdoors.

Meditation & Mantra

I am connected to all things.

Flowetry Prompts

How do I feel when I'm in nature?

January 9th

Set in Motion

We can set our life in motion by paying attention to all the good we have. As well as what we want to expand and flourish in our lives.

Meditation & Mantra

I live an expansive life.

Flowetry Prompts

What have I set in motion?
What am I looking forward to?

January 10th

Wildest Dreams

Dream as if there are no limits, and believe in your power to make them real.

Meditation & Mantra

Dream wild, believe.

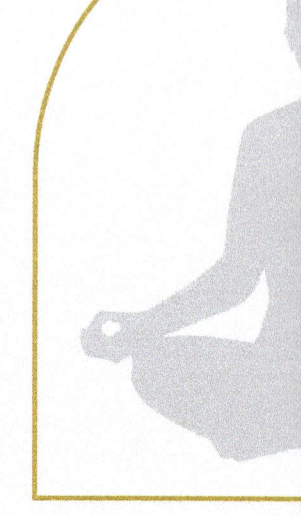

Flowetry Prompts

What are my wildest dreams? What am I going for?

January 11th

My Destiny

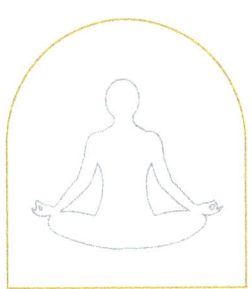

I am the queen of my own destiny, I take time to make my own path.

Meditation & Mantra

I walk my own path.

Flowetry Prompts

What small, intentional step can I take today to shape my own path and manifest my desires?

January 12th

I can and I will

I have what it takes, and I trust myself, I can & I will, just watch me.

Meditation & Mantra

I can.

Flowetry Prompts

Where do I see myself this time next year?

January 13th

Reinvention

Doing things you want to do but do it differently. Be open to change.

Meditation & Mantra

I am open to change.

Flowetry Prompts

What do I need to look at from a new perspective?

January 14th

Start Doing

What do I know supports me, yet I choose to not do it?

Meditation & Mantra

I choose me.

Flowetry Prompts

What can I start doing to support my hopes, dreams, body, mind & spirit?

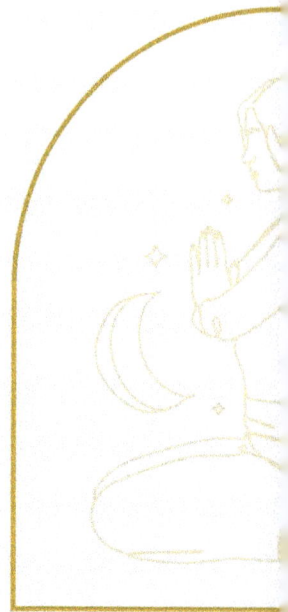

January 15th

Reliable

I can rely on myself. I am true to my word and I take inspired action.

Meditation & Mantra

I trust myself.

Flowetry Prompts

What benefits do I get from being true to my word?

January 16th

Dream, Create, Commit

First we dream, then we create it and we commit to the process.

Meditation & Mantra

I am a powerful creator.

Flowetry Prompts

What will I have created in 1 year? 3 years? 10 years?

January 17th

You are your answer

When you take time to study yourself and become self-aware you have the answer you are looking for.

Meditation & Mantra

I am my own answer.

Flowetry Prompts

If I knew the answer, what would the answer be?

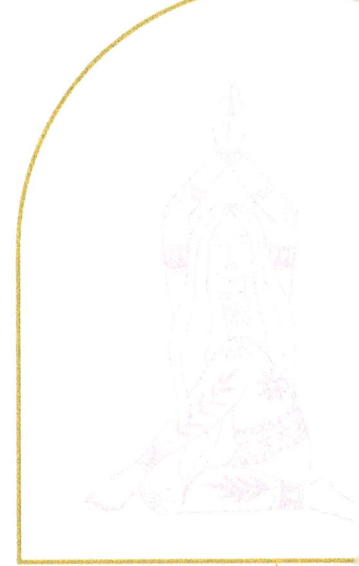

January 18th

Imperfection

One of the greatest hand brakes of all time. Perfection is in the eye of the beholder.

Meditation & Mantra

I am perfectly, imperfect.

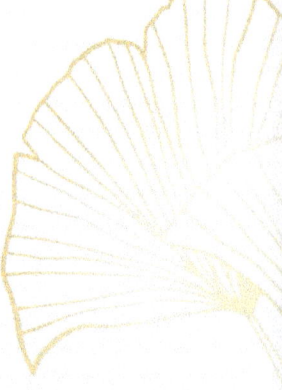

Flowetry Prompts

What imperfect action can I take today to move me closer to a feeling of contentment?

January 19th

Intuition

A knowing or understanding something without reasoning or proof.

Meditation & Mantra

I know what I know.

Flowetry Prompts

What do I know to be true?

January 20th

Self-Love

Today I will meet my own needs, avoiding the urge to please people.

Meditation & Mantra

It's safe to meet my own needs.

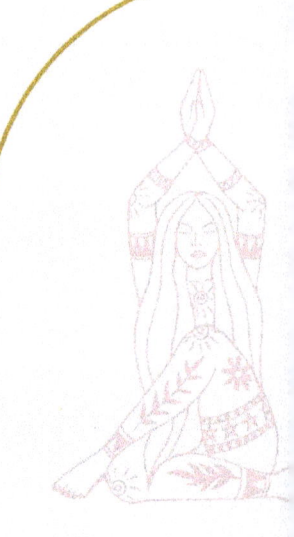

Flowetry Prompts

How can I take care of myself today emotionally, spiritually, physically?

January 21st

One Life

This is your life, and you get to choose! If you are displeased, take inspired action to make small changes. Its up to you!

Meditation & Mantra

I have choices, I can make changes.

Flowetry Prompts

What does it mean to have one life?

January 22nd

Out with the old and in with the new

Let the "old" go, whether it be objects, thoughts or emotions. Give them up. Let's make way for the new.

Meditation & Mantra

I welcome the new.

Flowetry Prompts

What's old and outdated that I need to let go of? What newness am I ready to invite in?

January 23rd

YOU

Yes, I'm talking to you! Get it together sista, the world needs your wisdom, creativity, love and your contribution. Step forward, it's your time!

Meditation & Mantra

I choose ME, the time is now.

Flowetry Prompts

What's my next step? How can I show up more?

January 24th

Sealed with LOVE

I lovingly seal off last year with love and appreciation for all I have learned and all I have grown.

Meditation & Mantra

Thank you past, I am wiser and stronger.

Flowetry Prompts

What wisdom came from last year's experiences?

January 25th

You only have NOW

Yep, its your time to Shimmer, you can and you will.

Meditation & Mantra

I can & I will.

Flowetry Prompts

What can I do and how will I do it? What's the next small step?

January 26th

How do you want to feel this year?

I Feel... No, we can't change what's happening around us all of the time, however you do get to choose how you feel.

Meditation & Mantra

I feel .....

Flowetry Prompts

How do I want to feel this year?

January 27th

Home

My home is my sanctuary, the energy lows freely and I am at peace.

Meditation & Mantra

My home is my sanctuary.

Flowetry Prompts

What I love about my home is? What needs to be decluttered in my home?

January 28th

Capable

I am more capable that I think I am. I'm unstoppable... Repeat.

Meditation & Mantra

I have what it takes.

Flowetry Prompts

Where in life am I capable?
Who is the most capable person I know?

January 29th

Wholehearted

To be wholehearted is to go after your deepest desires.

Meditation & Mantra

I am Whole and connected.

Flowetry Prompts

What does "Wholehearted" mean to me?

January 30th

See Clearly

Reignite old passions. New year and a new lens to see things clearly.

Meditation & Mantra

I see clearly.

Flowetry Prompts

What would I like to reignite in my life?

January 31st

Make it happen

We hold the keys to our own happiness and future. We are more powerful, smarter and resourceful than we think we are. Go for it!

Meditation & Mantra

I am resourceful.

Flowetry Prompts

What inspired action steps can I take to achieve my goals?

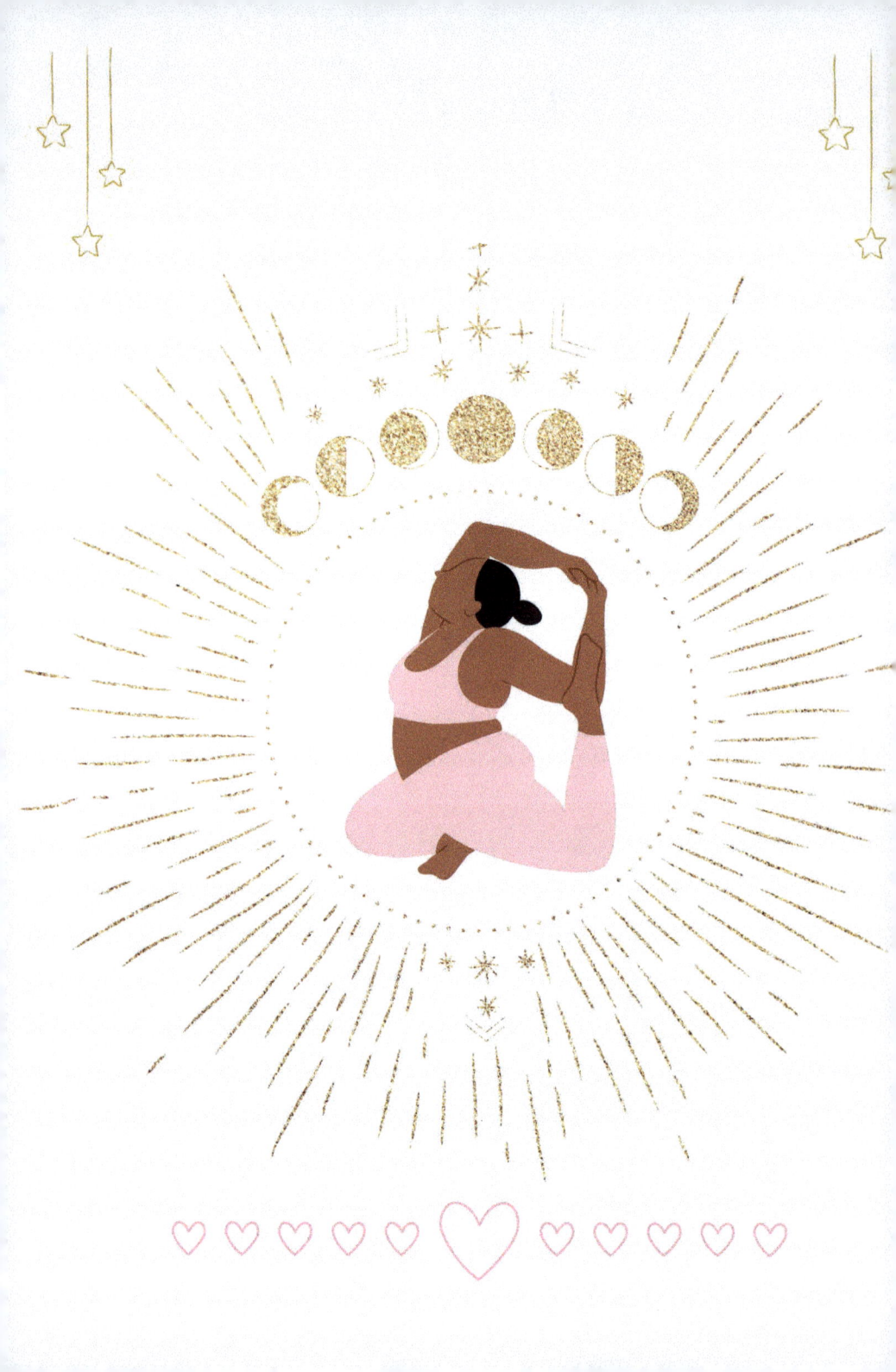

February

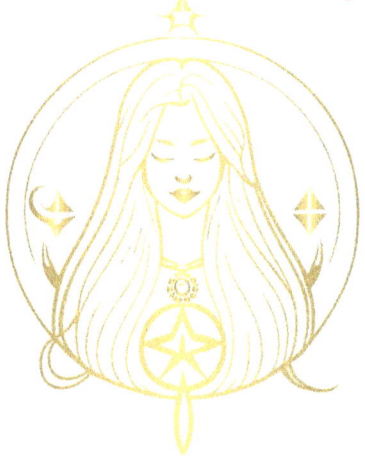

Commitment to Self

This month let's commit to none other than ourselves. You know, we often find it easier to dedicate ourselves to others or our daily grind, but what about our own beautiful selves? So, let's journey together through the art of self-commitment.

Let's embark on this introspective adventure, where we ask our hearts, "Am I my own cheerleader?" Are we standing by the promises we make to nurture our own growth and happiness? Imagine us, wise women, as gardeners of our souls, tending to the seeds of self-love and fulfillment.

So, let's make this month a symphony of self-devotion, a celebration of our commitment to our own radiant spirits. You've got the wisdom, the fire, and the grace – now, let's give ourselves the devotion we truly deserve.

February 1st

Commitment to self

I stay true to myself and I commit to me. I am exactly where I'm meant to be and I stay true to my path with a consistent energy flow.

Meditation & Mantra

I am consistent & committed.

Flowetry Prompts

What does consistent look like in my life? What am I committed to?

February 2nd

My heart's desire

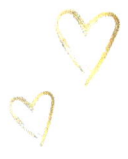

Imagine if you were consistent and committed to your heart's desire. Take a moment to listen to your heart.

Meditation & Mantra

I am committed to my heart's desire.

Flowetry Prompts

What's my heart's desire?
How can I commit to it?

February 3rd

Commitment to self-love & compassion

Self-love & compassion needs my presence. I learn more ways to express self-love and compassion. I am committed to the growth.

Meditation & Mantra

I am compassionately committed to me.

Flowetry Prompts

My commitment to self-love brings me what?

February 4th

This Year I will commit to more fun & play

I will make a commitment to myself, to make time for more fun & play. I will do things for the sheer joy of it.

Meditation & Mantra

I am playful & fun.

Flowetry Prompts

What does committed to play and fun look & feel like?

February 5th

My Purpose and passion needs my consistency to flourish

Tapping in purpose & passion takes a curious heart. Like a miner looking for gold he's consistent. Be the miner find your gold that's inside you.

Meditation & Mantra

I am the miner of my own gold.

Flowetry Prompts

If I were committed to my purpose what would that look like?

February 6th

Money, Prosperity, and Abundance

If there is one area in life that needs our commitment and consistency it's MONEY. When we are consistent & positive with our money it rewards us in more ways than one. Physically, spiritually & emotionally

Meditation & Mantra

I love my money & I love consistency.

Flowetry Prompts

What is my money goal this month?
When I'm consistent with my money goals I feel?

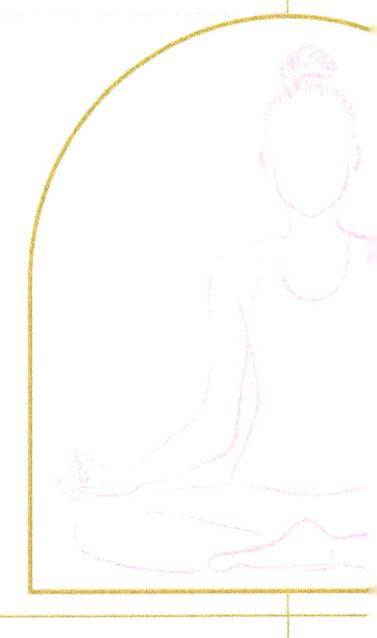

February 7th

Spirituality & Daily practice

When I'm committed & consistent with my daily practice, I reap so many rewards.

Meditation & Mantra

I am present.

Flowetry Prompts

What's my spiritual daily practice?
How does it benefit me?

February 8th

Holistic wellness

I take care of myself. My wellness is my priority and I reap the rewards for my commitment to my health.

Meditation & Mantra

I am radiant & vibrant.

Flowetry Prompts

What actions can I take to nurture my wellness?

February 9th

Home & Living Space

Our home is an extension of ourselves.

Meditation & Mantra

Ease & flow.

Flowetry Prompts

How can I make my home even more wholesome?

February 10th

Relationships & love

My heart is open and receptive to all the love that surrounds me.

Meditation & Mantra

I am love.

Flowetry Prompts

What is a loving relationship to me?

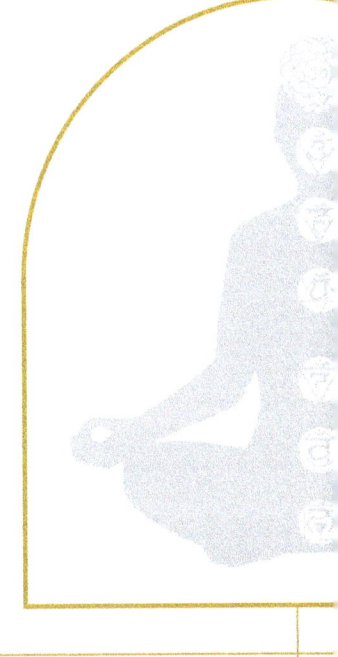

February 11th

You're worth it

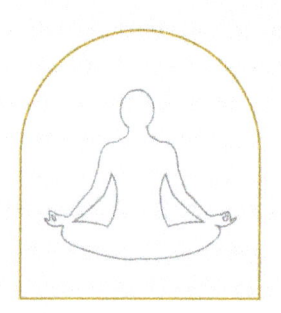

You are worth a hot cuppa, you are worth a 20 break, you're worth doing things for the sheer delight of it.

Meditation & Mantra

I am enough.

Flowetry Prompts

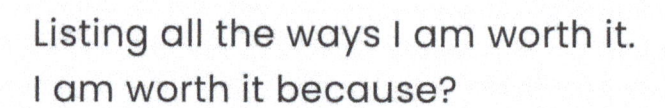

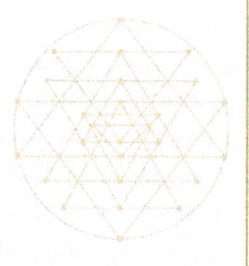

Listing all the ways I am worth it.
I am worth it because?

February 12th

Powerful presence

I'm too old to not own who I am. It's safe to be powerful in my presence.

Meditation & Mantra

I am a powerhouse.

Flowetry Prompts

Where do I feel most powerful?

February 13th

Tenacity

Be tenacious as a grey hair that doesn't want to be coloured. Sometimes you must stay true to who we are. Don't absorb what you don't want.

Meditation & Mantra

I am grounded.

Flowetry Prompts

What deserves my tenacity & why?

February 14th

Nerve of a Spiritual Warrior

It takes nerve to go after the dream, get out of your own way and stop s#%* talking yourself.

Meditation & Mantra

I have the nerve of a spiritual warrior.

Flowetry Prompts

Draw a spiritual warrior.
Describe a warrior.

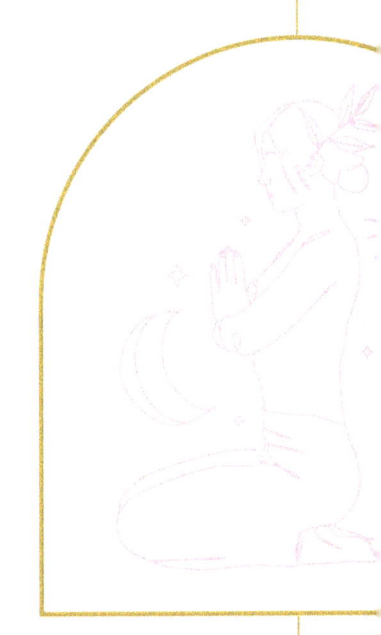

February 15th

Personal Power

The innate part of you knows what it takes and what the next step is.

Meditation & Mantra

I feel my personal power.

Flowetry Prompts

I feel my personal power in my body.
When I'm in alignment with my personal power I?

February 16th

Dependable

Can you depend on yourself? Are you showing up for you? We often want to depend on others but first we must start with ourselves.

Meditation & Mantra

I trust myself.

Flowetry Prompts

The actions I take to show myself that I am reliable are?

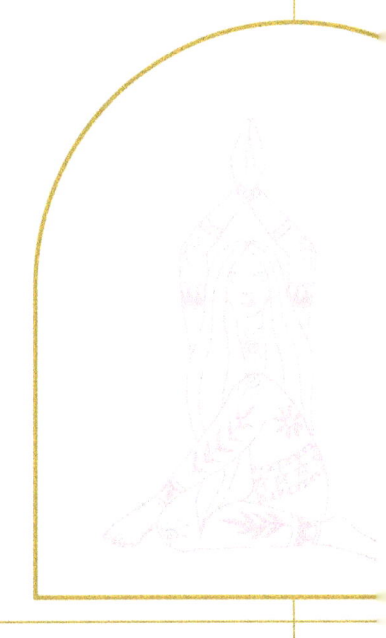

February 17th

Faithful to myself

I am faithful to myself, my goals and my dreams. I am committed & faithful!

Meditation & Mantra

I trust my faithful heart.

Flowetry Prompts

How can I strengthen my commitment to my goals & dreams?

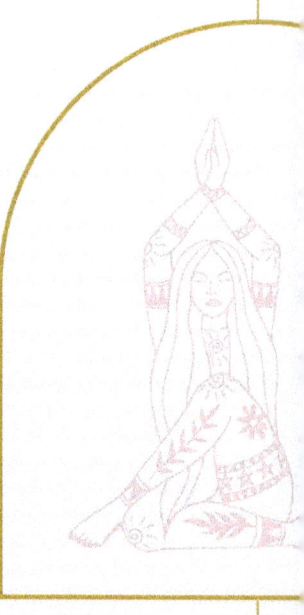

February 18th

The power of the spoken word

I say what I mean and mean what I say. Your words have power. Speak of only that you wish to have show up in your life.

Meditation & Mantra

I speak with love & kindness.

Flowetry Prompts

What am I not saying? How can I say it with a positive spin?

February 19th

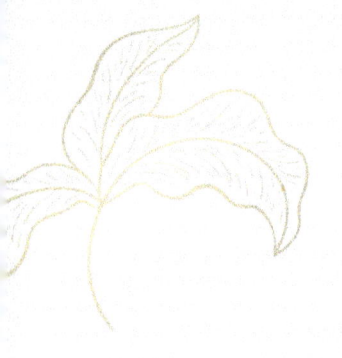

Devotion

I hold adoration for myself firstly and then to others.

Meditation & Mantra

I am devoted to myself.

Flowetry Prompts

What if I adored myself?
What would I do?

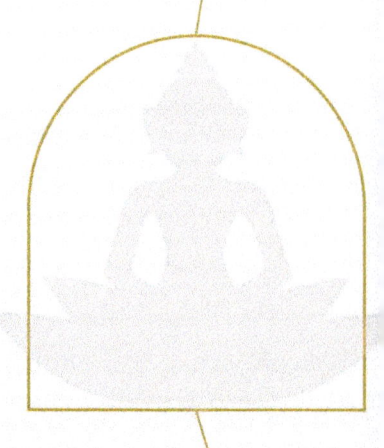

February 20th

Steady

Steady isn't always fast but steady is consistent.

Meditation & Mantra

I am unshakable.

Flowetry Prompts

Where in life am I steady? What does unshakable feel like?

February 21st

In tune

When I stay committed to my desires, I remain in tune with my heart.

Meditation & Mantra

I am in tune.

Flowetry Prompts

When I tune in, what does my heart say?

February 22nd

Rock

We all love a "Rock Person" in our life. Rock Person energy is committed & consistent.

Meditation & Mantra

I am consistent.

Flowetry Prompts

Where in life am I rock solid?
Who in my life is my rock?

February 23rd

What if

Imagine being committed & consistent in things that are important to you.

Meditation & Mantra

I am committed.

Flowetry Prompts

What if I raised my commitment & consistency to myself? What would happen?

February 24th

Have your own Back

Having your own back will change everything. You are everything you need.

Meditation & Mantra

I have my own back.

Flowetry Prompts

Having my own back means what?

… *February 25th*

Positive Determination

Determination in a positive light brings a personal power that is to be celebrated.

Meditation & Mantra

I am positively determined.

Flowetry Prompts

What area of your life need Positive Determination and why?

February 26th

Grit

Sometimes it isn't all rainbows and popsicle stands; it takes backbone and grit.

Meditation & Mantra

I have a backbone.

Flowetry Prompts

When was the last time I applied grit in my life? What was the positive outcome?

February 27th

Spunk and bedazzle

Sometimes it take a bit of spunk to make it happen. Be bold, be brave we need YOUR SPUNK.

Meditation & Mantra

I love being fully expressed.

Flowetry Prompts

When am I my Spunkiest? Who brings out all parts of me?

February 28th

You have already climbed a mountain

My love, no doubt you have already climbed a mountain or two, maybe even got stuck at the top or bottom from time to time. But you kept going.

Meditation & Mantra

I am capable.

Flowetry Prompts

What am I most proud of overcoming? Where am I most capable in my life?

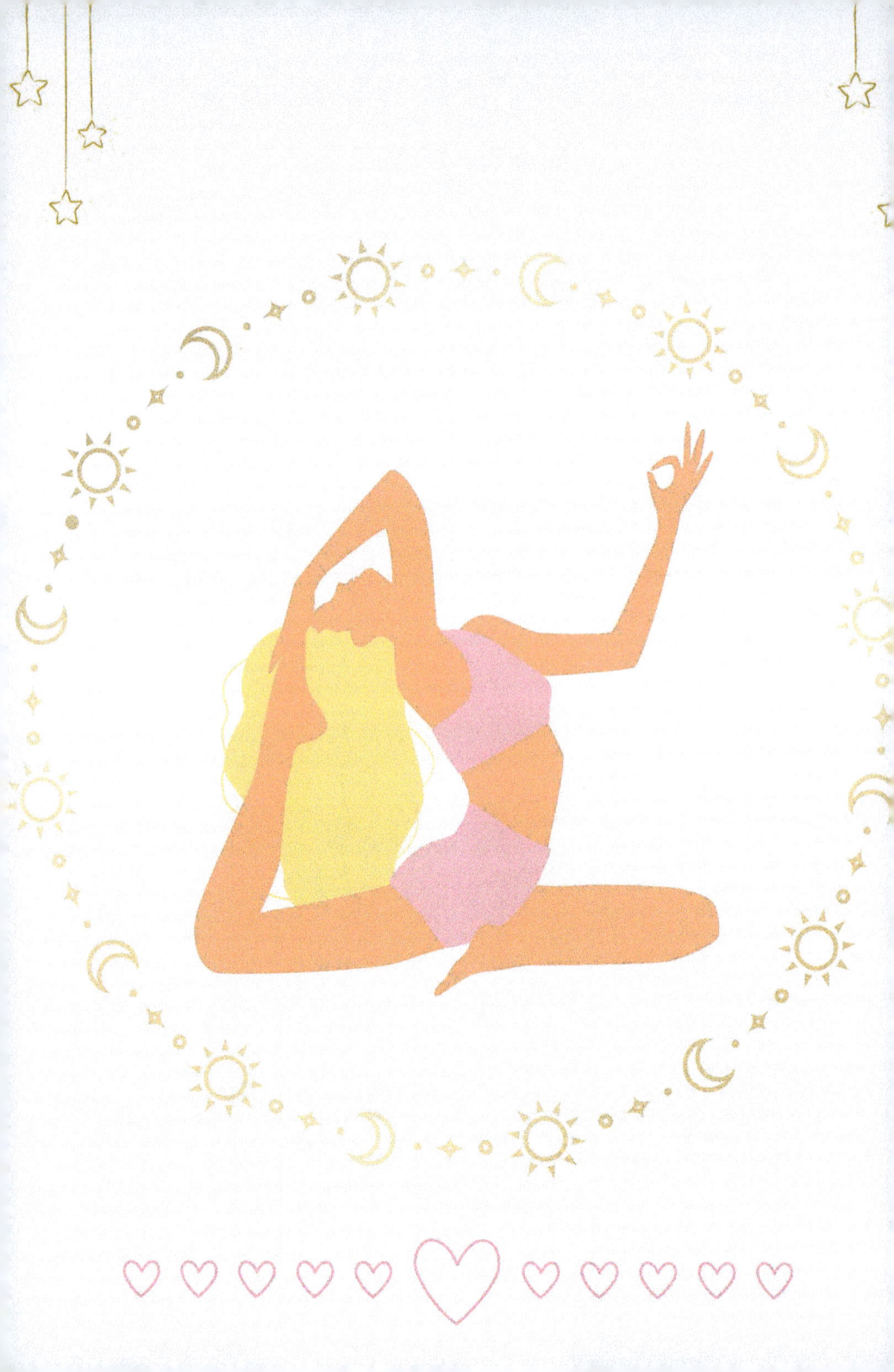

March

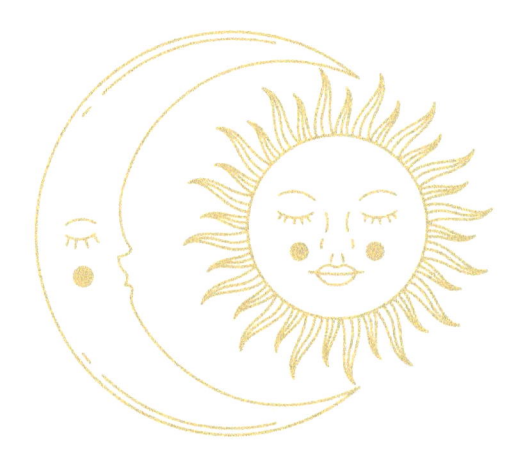

Self love & Compassion

A daily prayer:

Bring hands to heart center Anjali Mudra. Take prayer hands to third eye today I trust my intuition I know what I know. Bring prayer hands to lips today I'm impeccable with my words firstly and to others. Take prayer hands to heart center, today i do all things with love, kindness and compassion firstly to myself and then to others. The divine light in me sees and honours the divine light in you. Namaste

March 1st

It can wait just 1 hour

Your to do list will never be done, the washing basket will only be empty for an hour if you're lucky, there will always be a cupboard that needs cleaning- It can all wait. But your hot cuppa won't. Sit and enjoy.

Meditation & Mantra

I only have NOW.

Flowetry Prompts

What can wait?
What's a priority & why?

March 2nd

You can't give away what you don't have

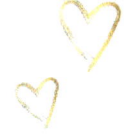

If you don't have peace, you can't give it away. If you don't love who you are, it's hard to fully love another, as you will never feel worthy. Start with YOU.

Meditation & Mantra

I am worth it.

Flowetry Prompts

Making a list of all the things I love about myself, from the way I look to personality qualities.

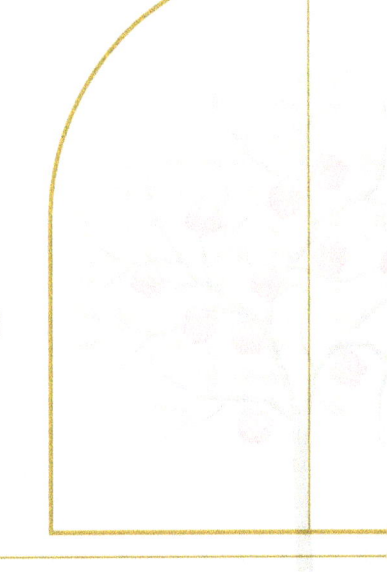

March 3rd

Have a Day to yourself

When was the last time you had a solo day all to yourself?

Meditation & Mantra

I love myself.

Flowetry Prompts

If I plan a solo day to myself, what would I do? Where would I go? How does it feel?

March 4th

Emotional Wellbeing

Emotional wellbeing needs to be on the top of your list. If you ain't good no one's good.

Meditation & Mantra

I am gentle to myself.

Flowetry Prompts

Focusing on my emotional wellbeing, what do I need? what support can I ask for?

March 5th

Physical Wellbeing

Your body is worth treating like a goddess.

Meditation & Mantra

I am here, here in my body, and all is well.

Flowetry Prompts

Writing a love letter to my body, telling her all the things I love about her and cherishing what she can do.

March 6th

Spiritual Well being

You get to define what spiritual well being is for you. You know how it feels and what the connection feels like.

Meditation & Mantra
I am connected.

Flowetry Prompts

Defining spiritual wellbeing in my own words.
What's my spiritual practices?

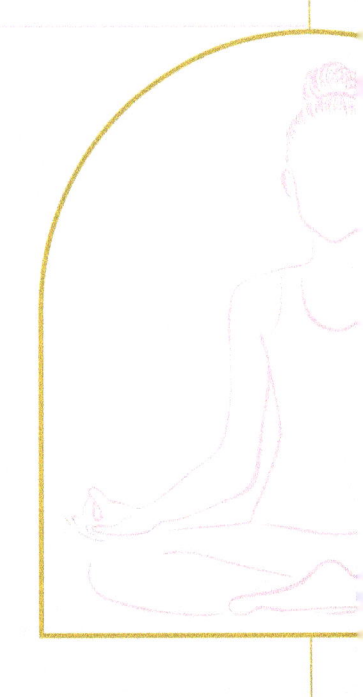

March 7th

Self-Compassion

I am compassionate, kind and joyful, firstly to myself and then to others.

Meditation & Mantra

I am compassionate with myself & others.

Flowetry Prompts

Where do I need to show myself more compassion?
Where do I need to show others more compassion?

March 8th

Don't save it wear it

If you are saving that new dress, top or pants for somewhere nice enough to wear it, stop it!

Meditation & Mantra

I'm worth it.

Flowetry Prompts

Why do I hold back on treating myself nicely?

March 9th

Do it now, as later may never arrive

Go for it, do it, you got this, your time is now.

Meditation & Mantra

I am present and ready.

Flowetry Prompts

What am I putting off? What do I want to pursue?

March 10th

Only one opinion matters

Your opinion is the only one that matters. Be proud of who you are and what you have created.

Meditation & Mantra

I am proud of who I am.

Flowetry Prompts

Writing a list of all the things I am proud of and why.

March 11th

You have done hard things and survived

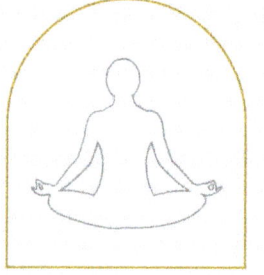

So far you have survived your worst day ever. You can handle hard things.

Meditation & Mantra

I have strength and courage.

Flowetry Prompts

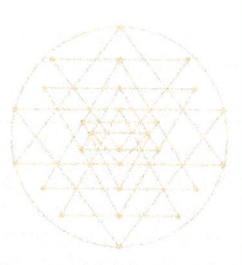

What have I overcome and how does it feel?

March 12th

Take a load off

There is no need to carry the weight of the world on your shoulders, we will let someone else do that.

Meditation & Mantra

It's safe to let go.

Flowetry Prompts

Asking my shoulders what they are carrying and why. Asking them kindly to let go.

March 13th

Fully Expressed

Showing up fully expressed and feeling free.

Meditation & Mantra

It's safe to be myself.

Flowetry Prompts

How do I like to fully express myself?

March 14th

Wonderful things are happening for me too

From time to time we may find ourselves feeling envious of another perceived opportunities. Remember wonderful things are happening for YOU too.

Meditation & Mantra

Wonderful things are happening.

Flowetry Prompts

What wonderful things are & have happened to me?

March 15th

I Don't Chase, I Align & Attract.

There is no need to chase or force, all I need to do is align and attract.

Meditation & Mantra

I attract my heart's desire.

Flowetry Prompts

What am I chasing?
What am I attracting?

March 16th

Rise with confidence

I rise up to meet life's challenges with calm & confidence.

Meditation & Mantra

I am calm & confident.

Flowetry Prompts

Where do I rise with confidence in my life? How does it feel?

March 17th

Inner Beauty

My inner beauty shines through, it's safe to be seen.

Meditation & Mantra

It's safe to be seen.

Flowetry Prompts

How can I shine today?
Where can I shine today?

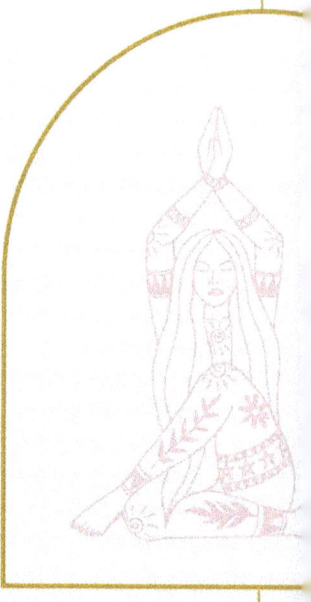

March 18th

Universal Protection

The universe protects and nurtures me. I am taken care of in more ways than I can imagine.

Meditation & Mantra

The universe protects me.

Flowetry Prompts

How does the universe protect me?
How does it feel?

March 19th

I draw on my inner wisdom

When I am confident and focused, my voice of wisdom guides me.

Meditation & Mantra

I welcome my voice of wisdom to speak to me.

Flowetry Prompts

Asking my voice of wisdom any question I want an answer to.

March 20th

My Glorious Body

My body is a glorious work of wonder.

Meditation & Mantra

My body is wonderful.

Flowetry Prompts

Giving kudos to my glorious body for all she has done for me.

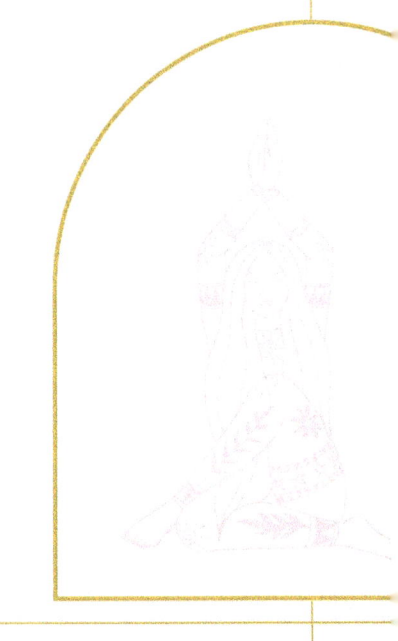

March 21st

Let Go

In any given moment you are free to let go. Let go of your past, let go of the future. You are here now.

Meditation & Mantra

I let go.

Flowetry Prompts

What do I need to let go of in the past?
What do I need to let go of in the future?

March 22nd

Let things flow

I allow life's energy to flow through me.

Meditation & Mantra

I allow flow.

Flowetry Prompts

What in my life is flowing and why?
What's NOT flowing and why?

March 23rd

My Essence

I am the essence of love, strength & courage.

Meditation & Mantra

I am love, strength & courage.

Flowetry Prompts

Love is?
Strength is?
Courage is?

March 24th

Be your own Hero & Heroine

I am heroic, sometimes in the smallest of ways and sometimes in a mighty way.

Meditation & Mantra

I am heroic.

Flowetry Prompts

I am my own hero/heroine because?

March 25th

Action with purpose and clarity

I know when to take action and when not to take action. My intuition is my greatest gift.

Meditation & Mantra

I listen to my intuition.

Flowetry Prompts

Allowing my intuition to guide me. Do I need to take action? Do I need clarity?

March 26th

I am supple in my mind & body

Being supple in my mind and body serves me well. I am open to other people's ideas and opinions.

Meditation & Mantra

I am supple & flexible.

Flowetry Prompts

Where do I need to be more flexible in life?
How does flexible feel?

March 27th

I Release all perceived obstacles

Obstacles in your way challenge your belief around perceived obstacles. Are you your obstacle?

Meditation & Mantra

I am free to move forward.

Flowetry Prompts

What is my biggest obstacle and why?
Did I create it?

March 28th

I give myself permission

Today, I give myself permission to go within and reenergize my body, mind & soul.

Meditation & Mantra

I am reenergized.

Flowetry Prompts

How can I reenergize today?

March 29th

Radiate Happiness

I radiate happiness and love everywhere I go, and it is returned to me.

Meditation & Mantra

I am happiness & love.

Flowetry Prompts

What do I want to radiate to the world?

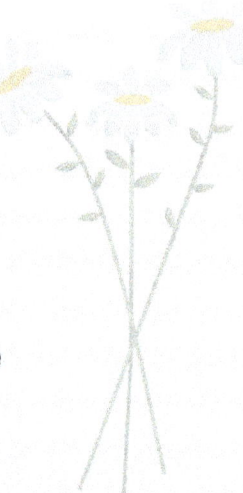

March 30th

I Receive

I receive goodness, I receive kindness, I receive love, I receive joy.

Meditation & Mantra

I am open.

Flowetry Prompts

What am I open to receiving?

March 31st

Breathe in breathe out

I inhale joy & happiness & exhale stress and negativity.

Meditation & Mantra

I breathe in joy & happiness.

Flowetry Prompts

What do I choose to inhale?
What do I choose to exhale?

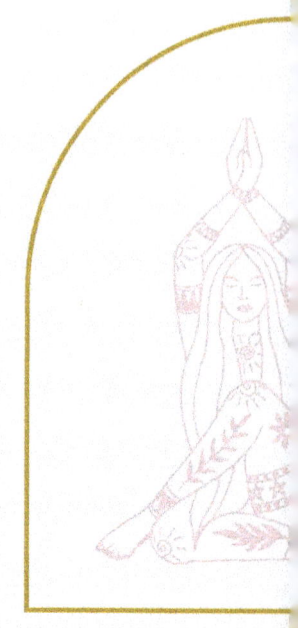

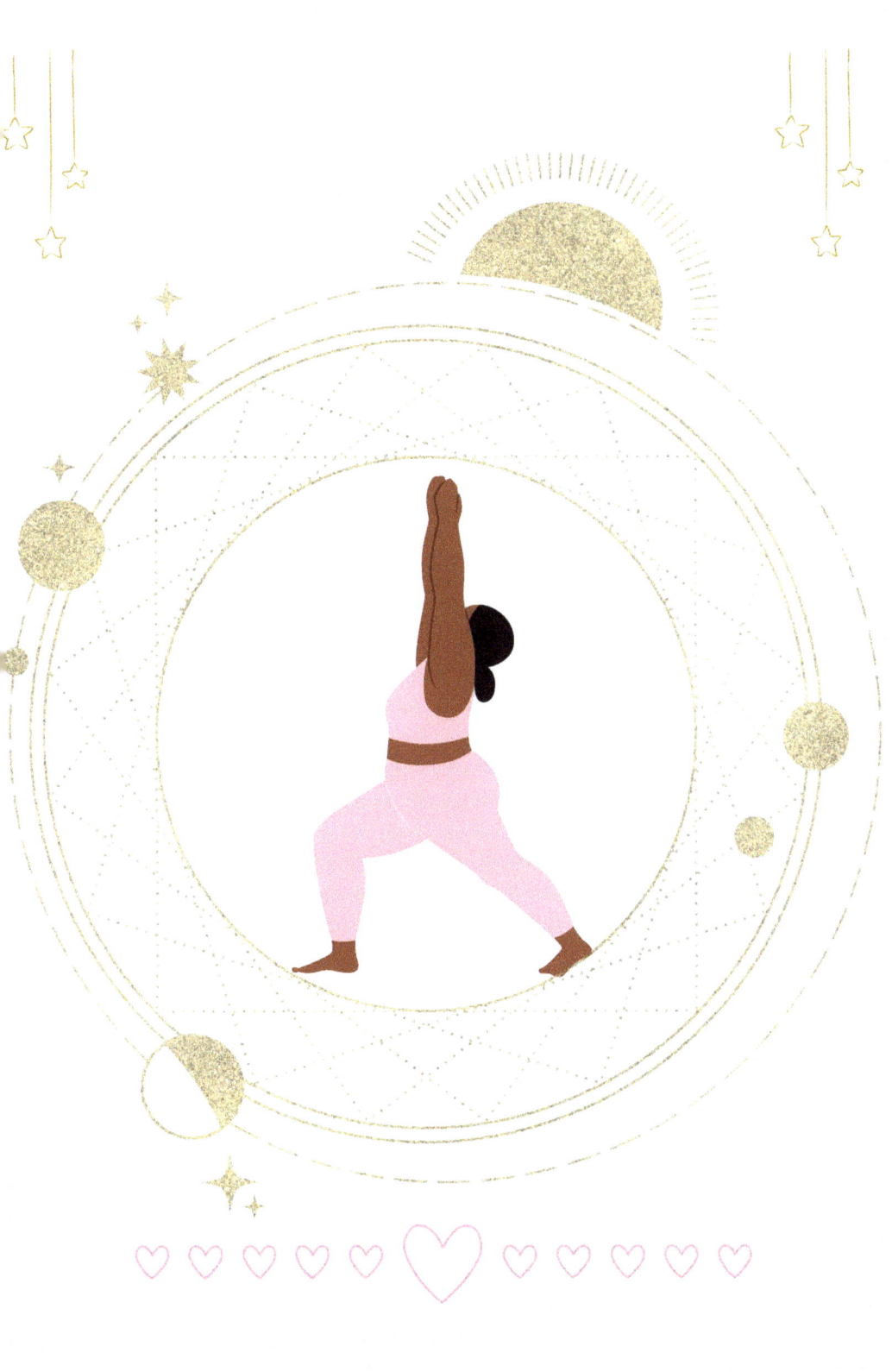

April

Purpose & Passion

In the quiet depths of my being, I find solace in the knowledge that my purpose and passion are not mere accidents, but a sacred choice I have the privilege to make. Yes i have many gifts and talents but my purpose and passion is a deep calling and wild horses couldn't stop it. Every step on this journey is a choice to heed the call of my soul, to embrace it with unshakable faith. I trust that I am precisely where I am meant to be, guided by divine synchronicity and surrounded by souls with whom I share a profound connection.

April 1st

Passionate Living

When wild horses couldn't stop you, you feel passionate and present.

Meditation & Mantra

I am living a passion filled life.

Flowetry Prompts

What couldn't wild horses stop me from doing?

April 2nd

Purposeful living

Living a purpose-driven life can harness endless energy to keep us on track.

Meditation & Mantra

I am living a purpose filled life.

Flowetry Prompts

What gives me a feeling of purpose?
Who do I know that is living a life of purpose?

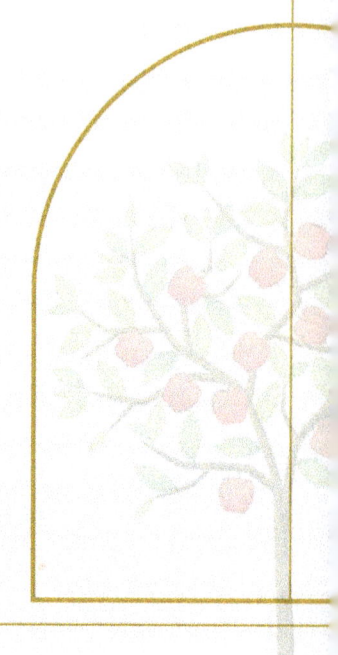

April 3rd

Your words Inspire

The words you speak firstly inspire YOU and then others.

Meditation & Mantra

I am inspired.

Flowetry Prompts

Who inspires me?
What inspires me?

April 4th

Daydream

To daydream and imagine a passionate, purposeful life is to bring joy right into your heart.

Meditation & Mantra

I feel passionate & purposeful.

Flowetry Prompts

Sitting and daydreaming about my wonderful, purposeful, and passionate life. Then, writing it out like a story from the heart.

April 5th

The Perfect Day

Have you ever had one of those perfect days that is imprinted on your heart and in your mind?

Meditation & Mantra

I rejoice in who I am.

Flowetry Prompts

Writing out my most perfect day.
Who am I with and what am I doing?

April 6th

A Home filled with Passion

When you look around your home do you feel passionate and supported?

Meditation & Mantra

I feel passionate and supported.

Flowetry Prompts

What does a passionate home look & feel like?

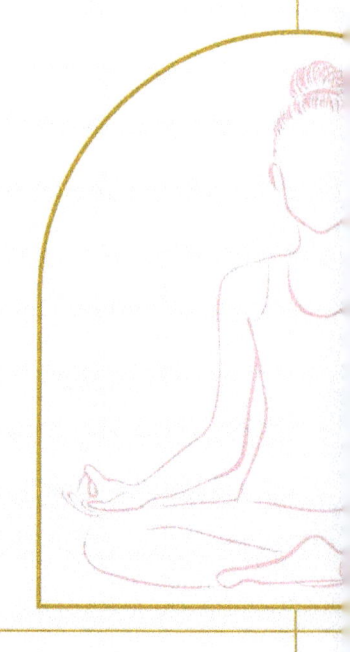

April 7th

Ambitious

Be bold, be ambitious, go after the things you want.

Meditation & Mantra

I am bold & ambitious.

Flowetry Prompts

Where in life am I ambitious?

April 8th

Aspiration

Aspiration, intention and actions towards my best self.

Meditation & Mantra

Today I aspire to be my best self.

Flowetry Prompts

What are my aspirations?
What are my actions towards my aspirations?

April 9th

BIG idea

How many beautiful big Ideas do you have?

Meditation & Mantra

I welcome big ideas.

Flowetry Prompts

What big idea do I have? What action can I take for it to manifest?

April 10th

Drift & float

Get in the bath and drift away, float, and allow the water goddess to whisper in your ear.

Meditation & Mantra

I am open and receptive to inspiration.

Flowetry Prompts

Get quiet, breathe and listen... Write down what you hear.

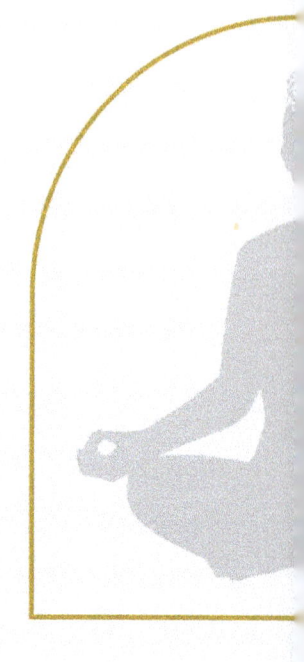

April 11th

Explore & Research

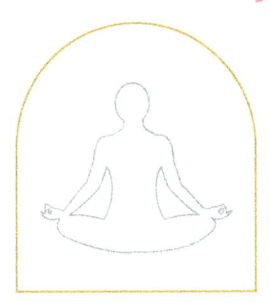

Explore & Research what you are passionate about.

Meditation & Mantra

It's safe to explore more of who I am.

Flowetry Prompts

What would I like to explore and research?
What am I curious about?

April 12th

Try something NEW

Be open to trying new things, you never know you may even like it.

Meditation & Mantra

It's a new day full of possibilities.

Flowetry Prompts

What would I like to try?
What possibilities lay before me today?

April 13th

I Feel Purposeful

I Feel purposeful, focused, determined and alive.

Meditation & Mantra

I feel purposeful in this moment.

Flowetry Prompts

Where in life am I purposeful, focused, determined and alive?

April 14th

I Feel Passionate

I feel passionate, enthusiastic & inspired.

Meditation & Mantra

I am Passionate.

Flowetry Prompts

Where in life am I passionate, enthusiastic & inspired?

April 15th

You choose your purpose

You get to choose what your purpose is, so now go and be brilliant at it.

Meditation & Mantra

I choose to be brilliant.

Flowetry Prompts

Choosing my purpose, what is it & how does it feel?

April 16th

It might scare you

Your purpose might scare the bejesus out of you and if it does, great you're right on track.

Meditation & Mantra

I own my purpose.

Flowetry Prompts

What part of owning my purpose scares me?

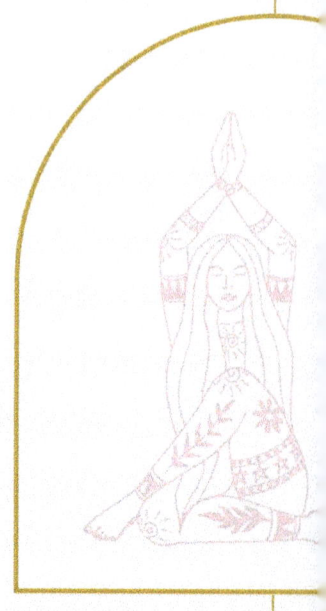

April 17th

Excitement

Feeling excited is a gift. Bask in the feelings of anticipation & excitement.

Meditation & Mantra

I am excited about my future.

Flowetry Prompts

What excites me?
What am I looking forward to in the future?

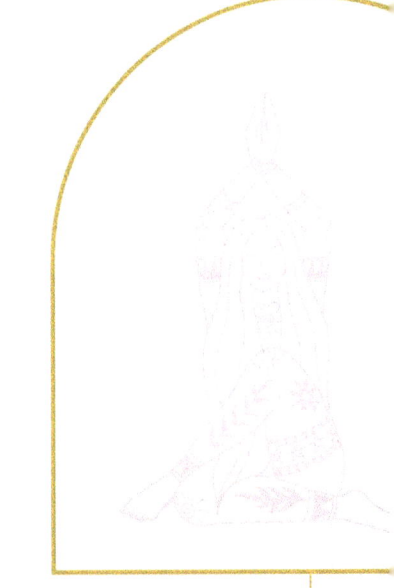

April 18th

Fire in my Belly

Fire in my belly, passion ignited and I'm going for it.

Meditation & Mantra

I am going for it.

Flowetry Prompts

What do I have a fire in my belly for? What am I going for?

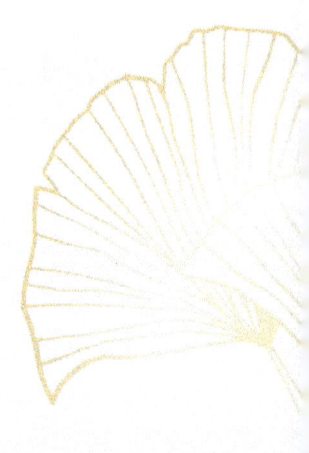

April 19th

Heartfelt Purpose

A purposeful heart is expanded and has a huge capacity to make positive change in the world.

Meditation & Mantra

I am on purpose.

Flowetry Prompts

Listening to my heart, what does it want me to know about my purpose?

April 20th

You were born original

There is no one else on this planet like you. You have a divine purpose because you were born.

Meditation & Mantra

I am original.

Flowetry Prompts

What makes me original?
What makes me, ME?

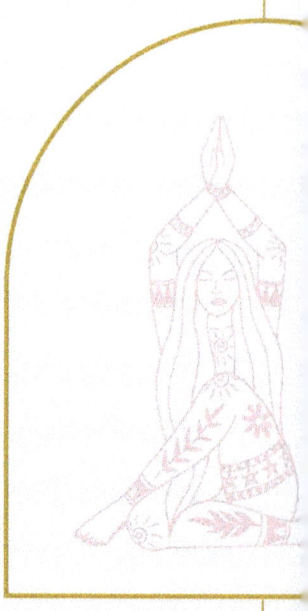

April 21st

Don't follow the rules

Don't follow the rules follow you heart, follow your passion, follow your purpose.

Meditation & Mantra

I follow my heart.

Flowetry Prompts

Where does my heart want to go? What does my heart want to do?

April 22nd

Break the Mould

Break the mould, bust out of the normal and the mundane, follow your passion.

Meditation & Mantra

I lead with a passionate heart.

Flowetry Prompts

What does the normal mould look like? What are the ways in which you have broken free from the mould?

April 23rd

Make your purpose be a priority

We all have obligations. Have you ever thought you have an obligation to make your purpose a priority?
The world needs you in the best version of YOU.

Meditation & Mantra

I prioritise my purpose, this is the best version of me.

Flowetry Prompts

What's the best version of me?
What priorities am I neglecting?

April 24th

Passion & Purpose Co-Create

Passion & Purpose are wonderful co-creators. They work in harmony with one another.

Meditation & Mantra

I am in harmony.

Flowetry Prompts

How can I bring my passion & purpose together?

April 25th

Encourage the blossoming of your passion

Just as you tend to your garden and give it love, tending to your passions and encouraging them to grow is to blossom.

Meditation & Mantra

I am blossoming.

Flowetry Prompts

Where am I blossoming in life?
What does blossoming feel like?

April 26th

Empty space

Sit and ponder, your purpose needs you to be still and create space.

Meditation & Mantra

I am still.

Flowetry Prompts

What does my purpose want me to know?

April 27th

Turn to Mother nature

When you step into Mother nature open your eye let the passion in you light up.

Meditation & Mantra

My passion is lit up.

Flowetry Prompts

When I spend time in mother nature how do I feel?

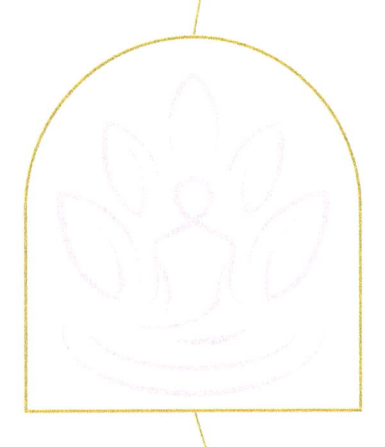

April 28th

You don't have to be good at it

Do it for the sheer fun of it. No pressure, be joyful & light.

Meditation & Mantra

I am joyful & light.

Flowetry Prompts

What is passionate fun?

April 29th

Your purpose whispers

Listen. Your purpose will whisper to you ever so quietly.

Meditation & Mantra

I am listening.

Flowetry Prompts

Listening to what the whisper is saying to me.

April 30th

Take the handbrake off

Go for it... Your purpose and passion are ready. Are you Ready?

Meditation & Mantra

I am ready.

Flowetry Prompts

Where do I need to take the handbrake off? What am I ready for?

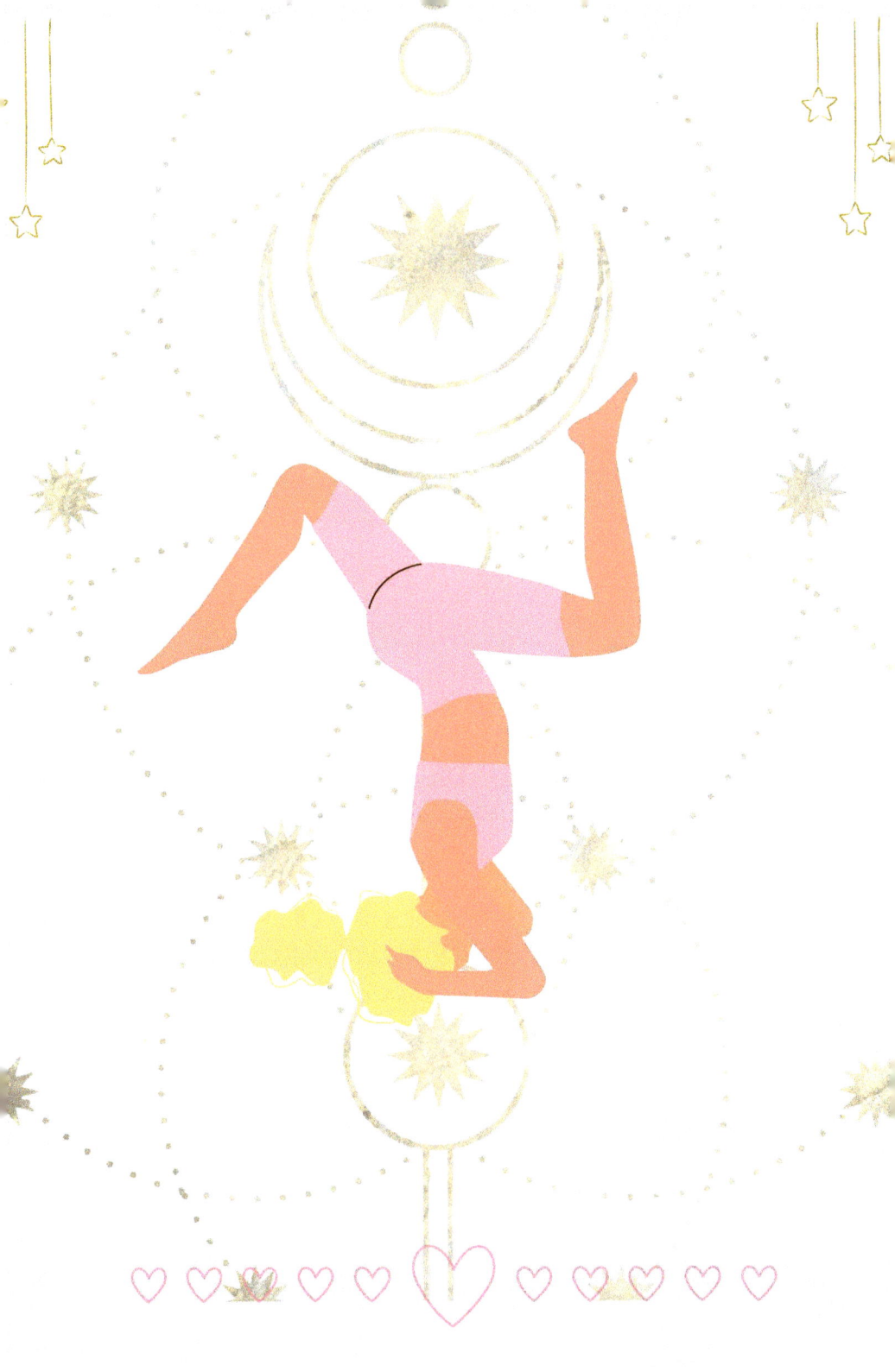

May

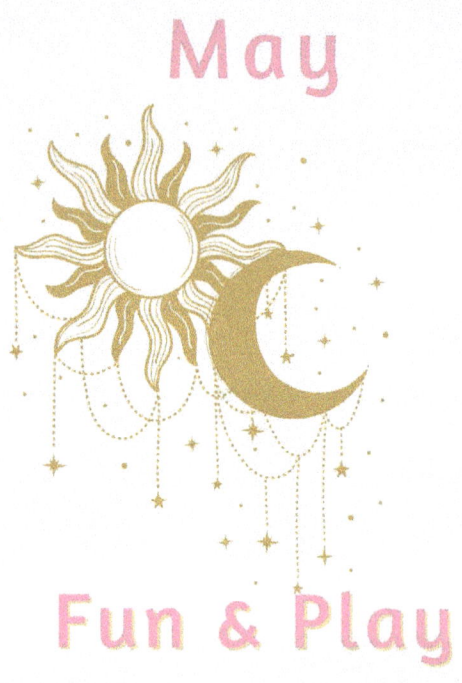

Fun & Play

Fun and play energize us, encouraging us to explore new possibilities and express ourselves creatively. Infusing fun and play into our daily routines can decrease our stress levels, uplift our mood, and heighten productivity. It's essential to discover and engage in activities that bring us genuine joy.
By prioritizing fun and play, we can establish a more adventurous, creatively fulfilled, and satisfying life. Let's commit to having more fun and injecting more play into our daily routines!

May 1st

Good old fashion fun

When I think of good old fashioned fun, I think of barn dancing, egg and spoon race, three legged race. Childhood memories.

Meditation & Mantra

My heart delights in play.

Flowetry Prompts

What is a fun memory from my childhood?

May 2nd

Playful

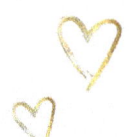

What's your idea of being playful?

Meditation & Mantra

I am playful.

Flowetry Prompts

Setting the timer for 7 mins, and seeing how many fun & adventure ideas I can come up with.

May 3rd

Adventure

Going on an adventure to explore and see new landscapes.

Meditation & Mantra

I am adventurous.

Flowetry Prompts

What adventure would I love to go on?

May 4th

New Experience

Stretch your mind and spirit with new experiences.

Meditation & Mantra

I am open to new experiences.

Flowetry Prompts

What would I love to experience and with whom?

May 5th

Mother Nature

When you are in sync with Mother nature, she supports your playful heart.

Meditation & Mantra

My heart is playful.

Flowetry Prompts

Where is my ideal place in Mother Nature? How do I feel?

May 6th

Create a playful environment

Creating a light & playful environment light me up in so many magical ways.

Meditation & Mantra

I am light & playful.

Flowetry Prompts

What do I love about my environment?

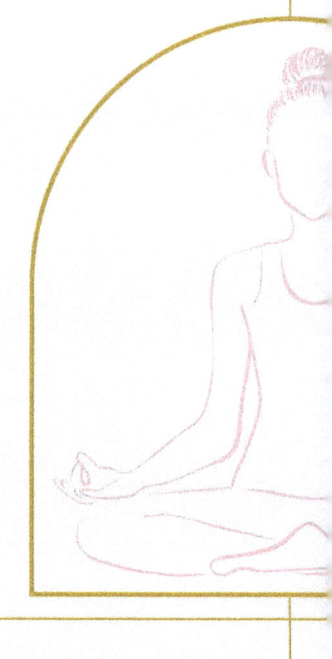

May 7th

Enhance your life

Enhancing your life with play, fun and adventure.

Meditation & Mantra

I am fun.

Flowetry Prompts

How can I enhance my life in the area of recreation?

May 8th

Hobbies

Hobbies allow your soul to play, and you don't even have to be good at it, just for the pure fun.

Meditation & Mantra

My soul is playful.

Flowetry Prompts

What are my hobbies? What hobbies would I love to take up?

May 9th

Your younger self

Your younger self loved to entertain themselves often in the simplest ways.

Meditation & Mantra

I am youthful.

Flowetry Prompts

Stepping into my youthful self, tapping into my playful inner child, what do I need and want?

May 10th

Schedule Playtime

Put it in your diary! It can't be all work and no play; life balance is a beautiful thing.

Meditation & Mantra

I am balanced and playful.

Flowetry Prompts

Planning out some playtime, what will I do? With who? What do I need to make it happen?

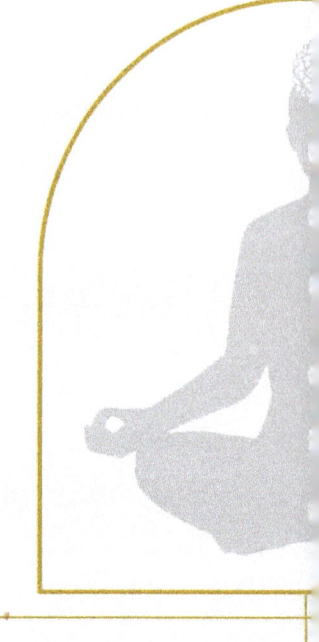

May 11th

My Mother, Margaret

The one who brought me into this world. She taught me to stand up for myself, go after what I want, and not to overthink it. Make it happen. My mother is a doer, a go-getter. She loves to give gifts and spoil me. But don't ask her opinion unless you want the truth. Thank you, Mum. I love you.

Meditation & Mantra

I am Fearless and Honest

Flowetry Prompts

What is your Favorite memory with your mother?

May 12th

Invite a friend

Enjoying the company of a fun friend.

Meditation & Mantra

I am filled with joy.

Flowetry Prompts

What would I love to experience with a friend?

May 13th

Solo

Take yourself on a solo play date, explore, relax and enjoy time to yourself.

Meditation & Mantra

I love my own company.

Flowetry Prompts

What would I love to do on my solo date? Where would I like to go?

May 14th

Play is essential

Play, joy & fun are essential to your mental & emotional wellbeing.

Meditation & Mantra

It's safe to be me.

Flowetry Prompts

When I have an adventure and play time how do I feel?

May 15th

Mood Booster

We are the creators of our own life and taking responsibly for our mood is an act of self love.

Meditation & Mantra

I am a powerful creator.

Flowetry Prompts

How can I boost my mood?
What do I like to do and with whom?

May 16th

Opening to creativity

Hobbies evoke more opportunity to express yourself creatively and explore new ideas and new perspectives.

Meditation & Mantra

I love to express myself.

Flowetry Prompts

Where am I most creative in my life? What are my favourite hobbies?

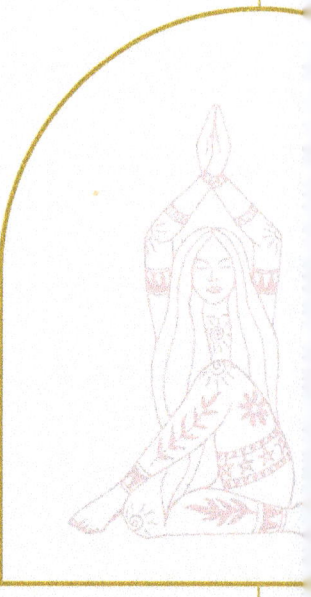

May 17th

Drop the responsibilities

Could you for one day drop all responsibilities and play?

Meditation & Mantra

I release control.

Flowetry Prompts
What responsibilities can I drop for 1 day? What would I do on the day?

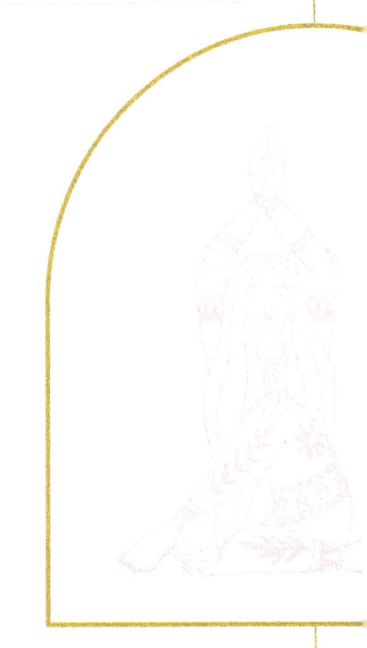

May 18th

Mix it up

You are not boring so stop acting like it! Today mix it up find new ways to express yourself.

Meditation & Mantra

I express who I am.

Flowetry Prompts

Who am I? How do I love to express myself?

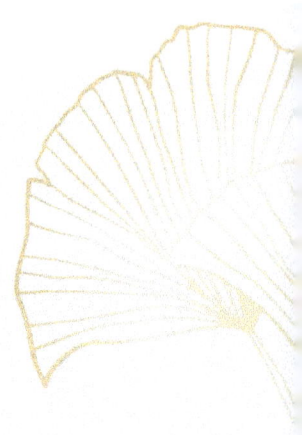

May 19th

Luminous

As, I start my day, I look to the sun to luminate me. I draw energy from its light. Shine bright today.

Meditation & Mantra

I am Luminous.

Flowetry Prompts

What do I draw energy from?
What drains my energy?

May 20th

Indulge

Indulge in whatever feels wonderful, it's fabulous for the soul.

Meditation & Mantra

I am worth it.

Flowetry Prompts

How do I like to pamper myself?

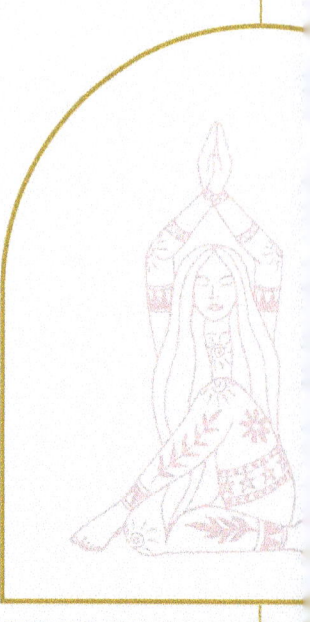

May 21st

Embrace your inner child

Release feelings of self-consciousness and allow yourself to be light and childlike. Remind yourself of what it was like to play without worrying about what others think and let yourself be fully immersed in the moment.

Meditation & Mantra

I embrace my inner child.

Flowetry Prompts

Stepping back in time to my 7 year old self, what would she like to do today?

May 22nd

Light-hearted friends

It's all about finding the right balance and surrounding yourself with people who are light-hearted, support and uplift you.

Meditation & Mantra

I am light-hearted.

Flowetry Prompts

Who are my light hearted fun friends & why?

May 23rd

Mind body & soul

Challenge yourself go on and adventure, expand your mind, body, and soul.

Meditation & Mantra

I am expensive.

Flowetry Prompts

If I were to challenge my mind, body & soul what would that look and feel like?

May 24th

Unique Places

There are so many unique locations around the world, be adventurous, visit the unusual.

Meditation & Mantra

I am ready to explore the world.

Flowetry Prompts

What unique lands and cultures would I love to explore? And with who?

May 25th

Stretch Yourself

You can stretch yourself and go to far away places and discover new territory.

Meditation & Mantra

I am ready to discover new things about me.

Flowetry Prompts

What stops me from stretching myself? What am I afraid of?

May 26th

What are you waiting for?

Your time is NOW, take the trip, go on the adventure, make time to play and explore.

Meditation & Mantra

It's my time to explore.

Flowetry Prompts

Setting a date, picking a location, allocating the money. I'm planning it. GO!

May 27th

Water Play

Water would have to be one of the most fun & playful elements. From waterfalls to the waves in the ocean.

Meditation & Mantra

My breath is like a wave in and out.

Flowetry Prompts

What are my favourite water memories? Pool? Beach? Waterfall?

May 28th

I Love my life

Fall in love with every part of your life, you are the main character.

Meditation & Mantra

I love my life.

Flowetry Prompts

Listing all the things I love about my life & why?

May 29th

More of it

More play, More happiness,
More Joy, More adventures.

Meditation & Mantra

I am ready for more.

Flowetry Prompts

What do I want more of?

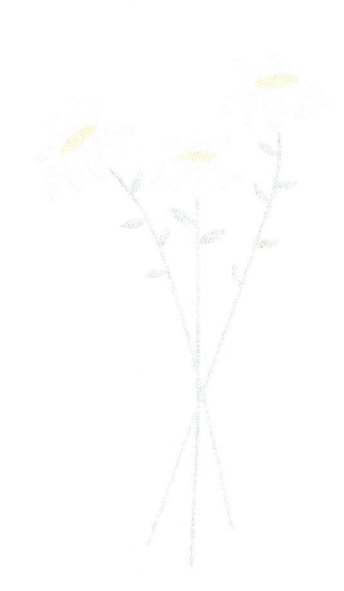

May 30th

Dreams are for free

Dreams are for free, write them down, daydream about them and then make them come to life.

Meditation & Mantra

My dreams will come true.

Flowetry Prompts

Writing down all my hopes & dreams.

May 31st

Light me up

I know what I lights me up and I choose to create more of this.

Meditation & Mantra

I am my own shining light.

Flowetry Prompts

What lights me up? My list of people, place and things that light me up.

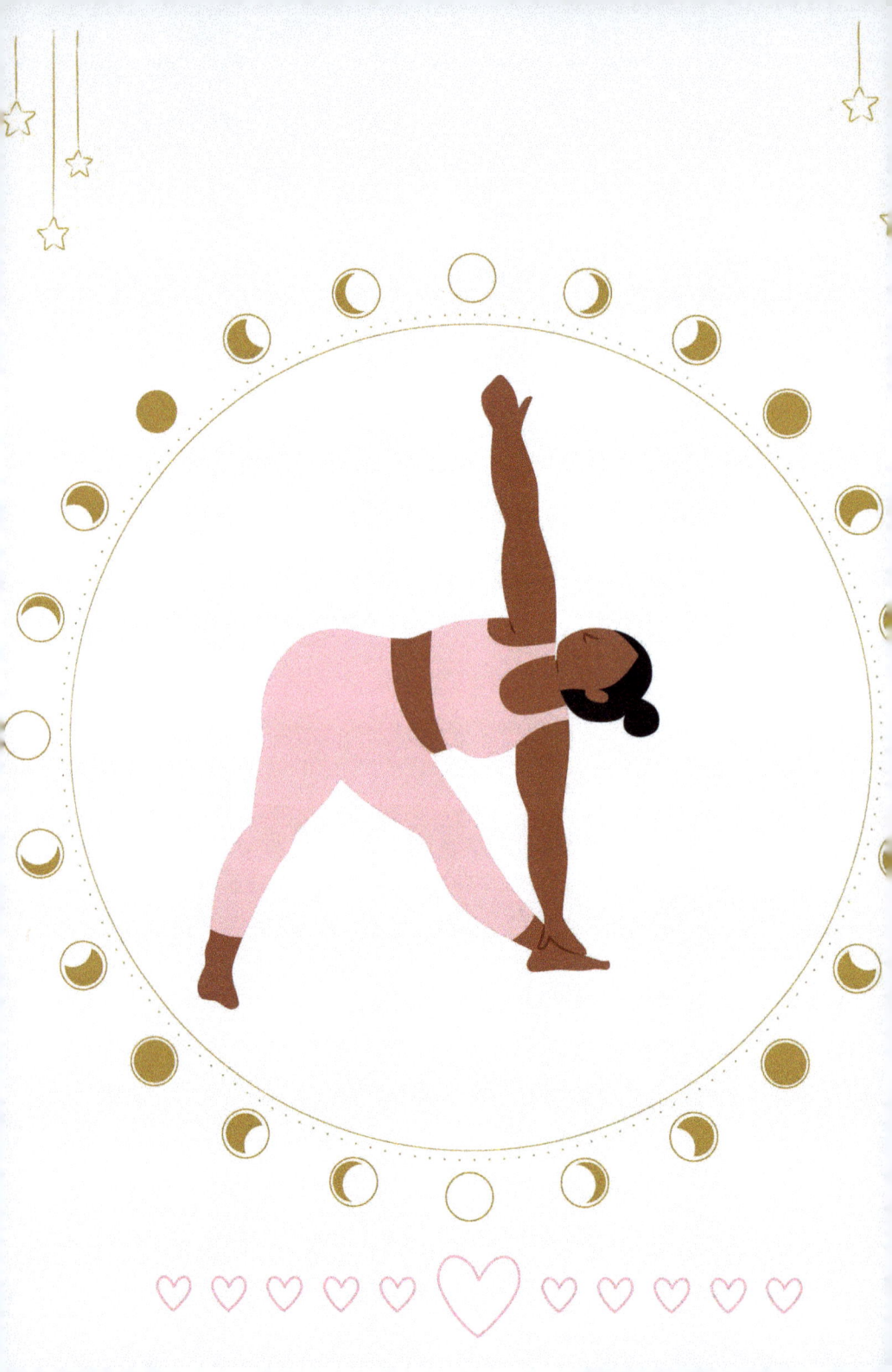

June

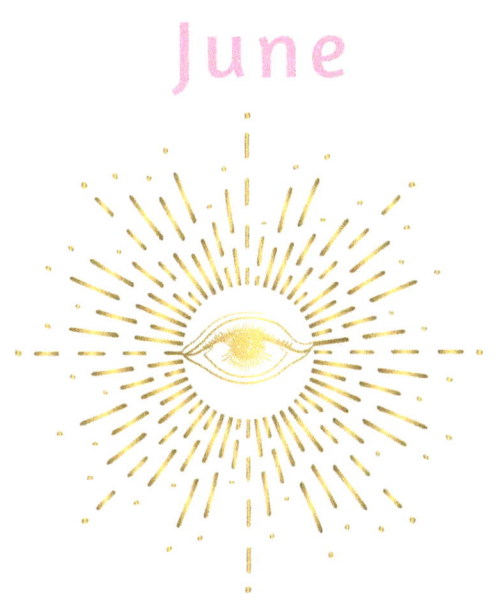

Money prosperity & Abundance

Money, abundance, and prosperity empower us, allowing us to experience financial freedom and security while also pursuing a purpose-driven life.

Incorporating a mindset of wealth and abundance into our daily lives can enhance our overall well-being, increase our confidence, and enable us to pursue our passions.

By opening up to money, abundance, and prosperity with a sense of purpose, we can establish a thriving life that goes beyond material wealth.

Let's commit to embracing a wealth-conscious mindset, integrating abundance practices into our daily routines, and seeking deeper meaning and fulfilment in all that we do!

June 1st

Prosperity is Everywhere

Prosperity is everywhere for me to witness. I watch and learn from mother nature.

Meditation & Mantra

I live in a prosperous world.

Flowetry Prompts

What has mother nature taught me about prosperity?

June 2nd

Money Grows on Trees

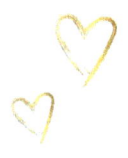

You may have heard the opposite growing up, but if you own an orchard, it's the truth.

Meditation & Mantra

Money grows.

Flowetry Prompts

Where have I grown in life? How can I grow my money mindset?

June 3rd

Love Affair with Money

Money and I love and respect each other. We have fun together and have a growth mindset.

Meditation & Mantra

I am in harmony with my money.

Flowetry Prompts

Writing a letter of gratitude to my money.

June 4th

Meaning of Bills

Bills are "Invoices for Blessings already Received".
How wonderful we get power & phone calls.. and then pay after we have had the enjoyment.

Meditation & Mantra

I bless all my bills with love.

Flowetry Prompts

How do I feel about receiving bills?
What's the positive?

June 5th

Open to More

Opening your mind and your heart to more, being open to the unexpected.

Meditation & Mantra

I am worthy of more financial flow.

Flowetry Prompts

Writing down all the reasons why I am open to more financial flow? How does it feel?

June 6th

Mindset of Prosperity

The universe is listening. What language around money and abundance do you need to shift?

Meditation & Mantra

In my prosperous mindset, I am powerful.

Flowetry Prompts

Inviting my mindset of prosperity to take the pen and write a future 12 months of growth and abundance.

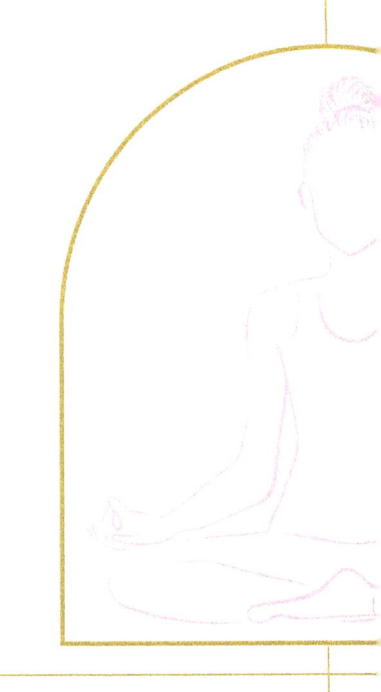

June 7th

Tell a New Story

From time to time, we get caught in telling a story of lack and scarcity.

Meditation & Mantra

Abundance and prosperity are my true nature.

Flowetry Prompts

Where do I feel lack or scarcity in my life? Now, let me flip this script and tell a new story of hope and positivity.

June 8th

First-Class Life

You are living a first-class life in so many ways. You just need to open your eyes.

Meditation & Mantra

I see abundance everywhere.

Flowetry Prompts

A big, beautiful list of all the amazingness I have around me, the seen and unseen.

June 9th

It's a Feeling

It's a feeling and only you can measure it! Abundance and prosperity are in the eye of the beholder. We all have our own interpretation.

Meditation & Mantra

I feel abundant & prosperous.

Flowetry Prompts

Today, I take time to acknowledge myself for all the goodness I have created in my life.
Writing a Thank You note to myself.

June 10th

Circulate it

Money is meant to be circulated.
It's a flow and a rhythm.

Meditation & Mantra

I am in rhythm with the
flow of money.

Flowetry Prompts

What does it mean to me to
be in flow and rhythm with
my money?
How does it feel?

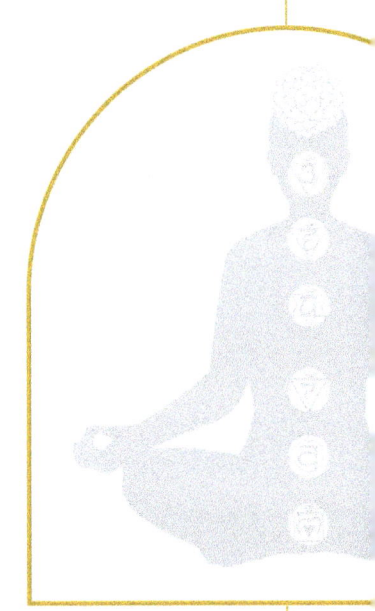

June 11th

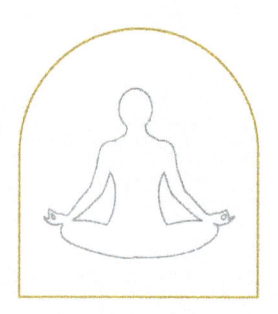

Order it

When you put your order in to the universe, only write down what you want - not the opposite.

Meditation & Mantra

I am ready to receive my order from the universe.

Flowetry Prompts

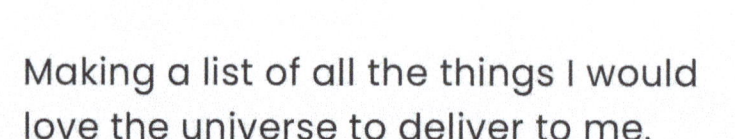

Making a list of all the things I would love the universe to deliver to me.

June 12th

Eyes Up Hearts Up

I love receiving signs from the universe that I'm on the right track, it's my job to pay attention and follow the signs.

Meditation & Mantra

I see the unseen.

Flowetry Prompts

What do I know for sure about my abundant life?
What does prosperity feel like?

June 13th

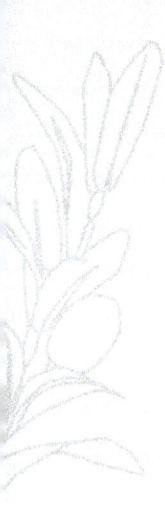

What would you do?

Imagine if money wasn't a consideration.

Meditation & Mantra

I am free.

Flowetry Prompts

If I didn't have to think about money, what would I do?
Where would I go?

June 14th

Priceless

The adventure, experiences, and relationships or connections can't be bought because they are priceless.

Meditation & Mantra

I am valuable.

Flowetry Prompts

Making a list of all the things in my life that can't be bought or have a price put on them.

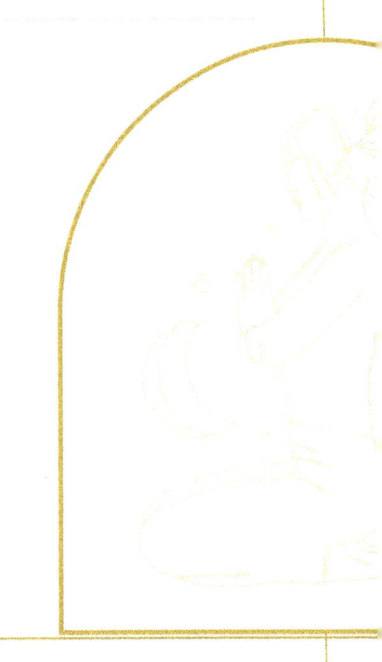

June 15th

Claim Your Power

You have the power to make as much money as you like.
Claim this power now.

Meditation & Mantra

I claim my power.

Flowetry Prompts

I have the power to create an abundant life, what's holding me back and why?

June 16th

Favour the Brave

Abundance and prosperity favours the brave.

Meditation & Mantra

Brave and Abundant.

Flowetry Prompts

What do I want to go after? Where could I be braver & more abundant?

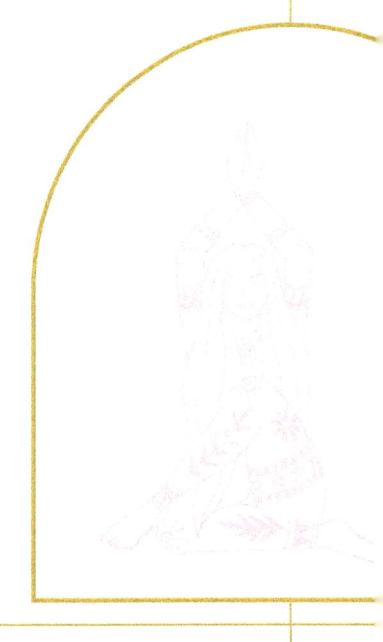

June 17th

Money Manager

When you take care of your money, your money takes care of you.

Meditation & Mantra

Ease and flow.

Flowetry Prompts

How do I take care of my money?
How does my money take care of me?

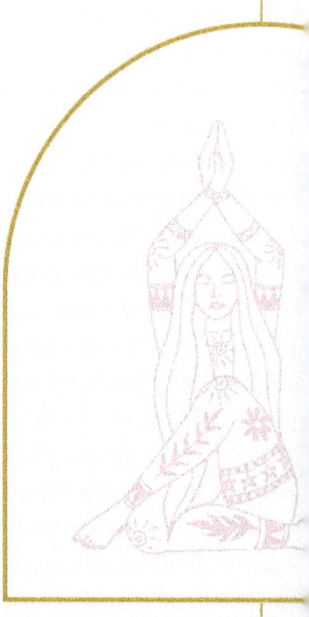

June 18th

Rich Life

Your life is a tale of highs and lows, wins and losses. Some may call it a full rich life.

Meditation & Mantra

I am Rich.

Flowetry Prompts

Writing about all the richness I have in my life.

June 19th

More Choices

What I love about money is that it gives me more options and choices.

Meditation & Mantra

I choose.

Flowetry Prompts

What choices do I have?
What options do I have?

June 20th

Money

Money — You can make it, you can create it, you can attract it, you can be given it, you can give it away, you can save it, you can spend it.

Meditation & Mantra

It's my choice.

Flowetry Prompts

What does money feel like to me?

June 21st

Money Romance

Money love story, how is your relationship with money?

Meditation & Mantra

I am love.

Flowetry Prompts

Writing my money a love letter.

June 22nd

Go for it

Your time is now, go for it, become obsessed with it, create it!
It's time to take the park brake off.

Meditation & Mantra

I am going after my dreams.

Flowetry Prompts

What am I obsessed with?
What do I want to create?
Where do I need to take the park brake off?

June 23rd

More than Enough

There is more than enough to go around. There is abundance and prosperity everywhere.

Meditation & Mantra

I see, I trust.

Flowetry Prompts

What do I have enough of in life?
What do I want more of in life?

June 24th

Affluence

Prosperity, Wealth, Riches, Privilege, Charmed.

Meditation & Mantra

I am.

Flowetry Prompts

What does affluence look and feel like?

June 25th

You Attract What You Feel

You attract what you feel.
I feel happy, wholesome, prosperous, and affluent.

Meditation & Mantra

I feel abundant.

Flowetry Prompts

How does it feel to be abundant and prosperous?

June 26th

Appreciate your Pennies

It's an equal energy exchange.
Love them and they will love you back.

Meditation & Mantra

I appreciate my pennies.

Flowetry Prompts

In what way do I appreciate my pennies?

June 27th

Consistently Abundant

I am consistent in my ability to attract abundance, prosperity, & affluence into my life.

Meditation & Mantra

I am consistently abundant.

Flowetry Prompts

What actions and thoughts do I practice - attracting more abundance, prosperity and affluence into my life?

June 28th

Positively Energised

I surround myself with positively energised people.

Meditation & Mantra

I am Positively Energised.

Flowetry Prompts

Making a list of positive energized people in my life, and why?

June 29th

Levelling Up

Level up, embrace growth, let it be easy.

Meditation & Mantra

I embrace growth.

Flowetry Prompts

When have I been outside my comfort zone and what did I learn about myself?

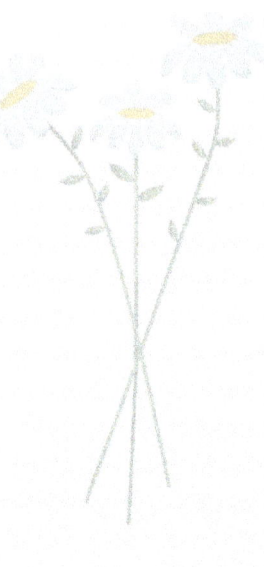

June 30th

Lighthouse

You are the provider of light for yourself and others.

Meditation & Mantra

I am the lighthouse.

Flowetry Prompts

Writing down three examples of how I have been my own answer and shining light.

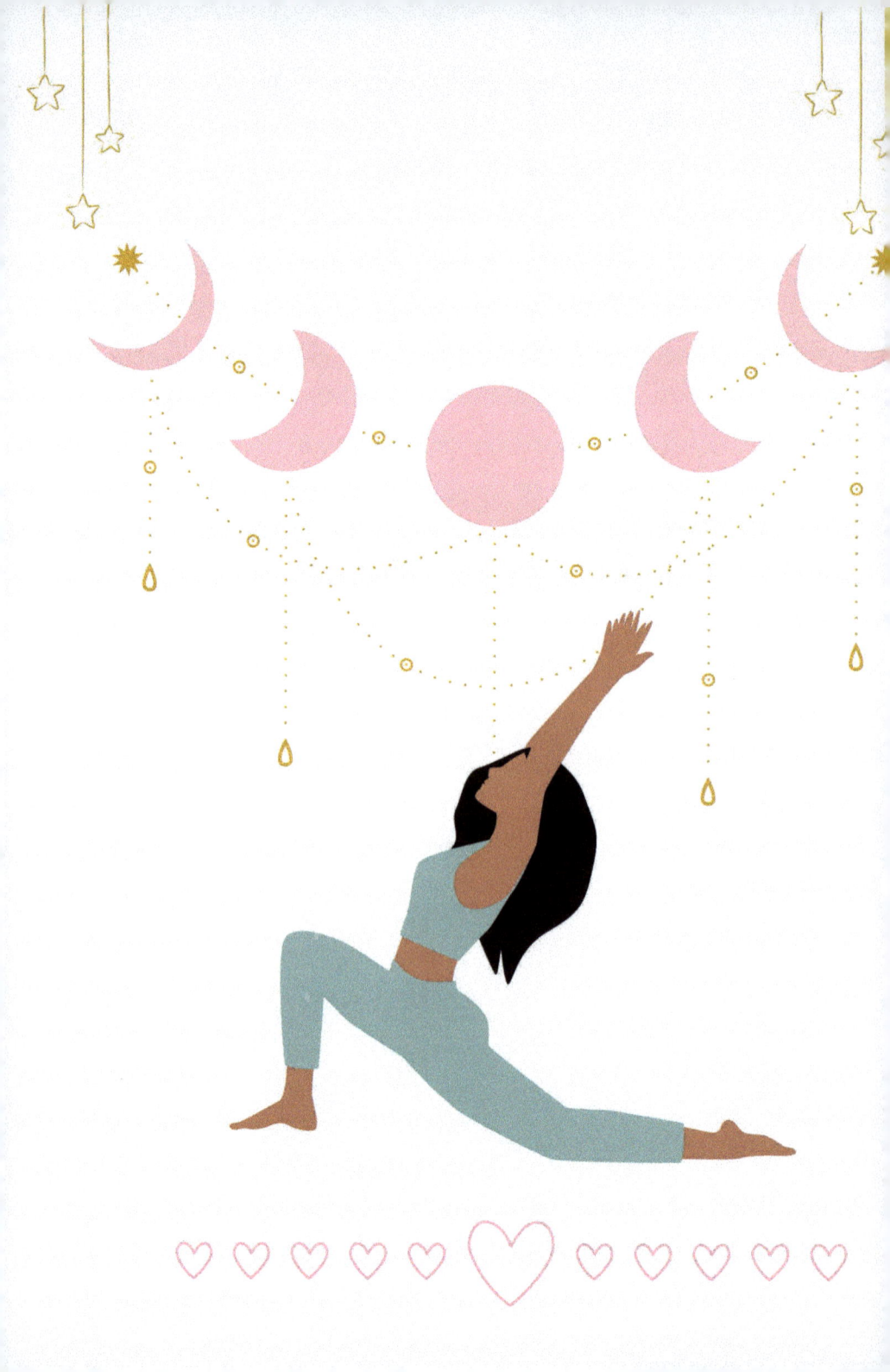

July

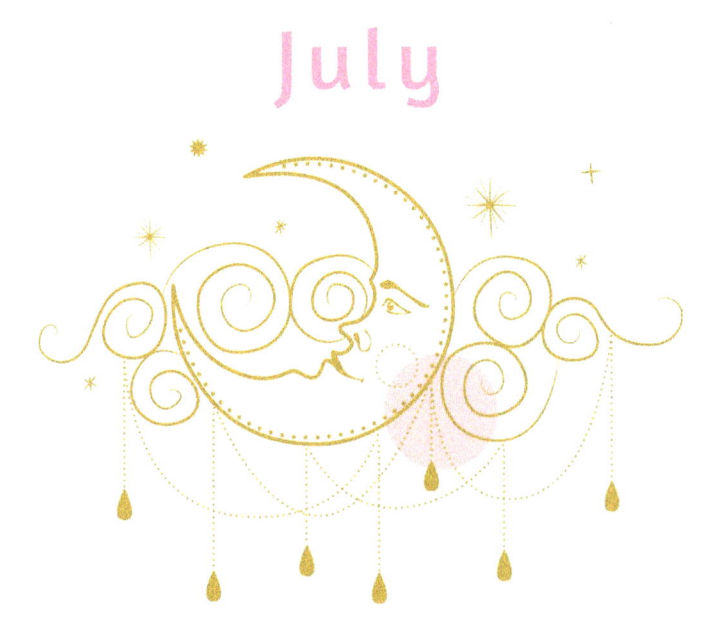

Spirituality & Daily Practice

Welcome friends! This July, we embark on a journey of spirituality, daily practice, and soulful rituals. Let's explore practices that inspires us, bring inner calm, and empower our souls.

- Embrace Daily Practice of your 21 Minutes of Morning Magic: Yoga, Mediation, journaling- let's discover ways to infuse intention and mindfulness into our daily lives.
- Create Soulful Rituals: Celebrate achievements, manifest dreams and find meaning through intentional rituals. From morning affirmations to visualizations, let's unlock transformation together

July 1st

Yoga

Yoga heals and reveals, the spiritual practice of yoga is to connect with yourself through breathe, meditation and movement.

Meditation & Mantra

So Hum (meaning- I am that)

Flowetry Prompts

What is my relationship with yoga? How do I feel about yoga?

July 2nd

What do you feel like

Tune into your body and how you feel to identify what you need at this moment.

Meditation & Mantra

I meet my own needs.

Flowetry Prompts

What does my body need today? How does my body feel today?

July 3rd

Small steps daily

Small steps daily cover a lot of ground over a year.

Meditation & Mantra

I create only good in my life.

Flowetry Prompts

What small daily steps can I take? Am I committed to these steps and why?

July 4th

Self-Love affirmations

Creating your own affirmations that light you up and inspire you.

Meditation & Mantra

I love my authenticity.

Flowetry Prompts

Set the time for 7 mins and write a list of self-love affirmations.

July 5th

Sacred Mindful Bathing

Using your daily shower/bath as a meditation. Dropping your favourite essential oil on the shower floor or in bath, lighting a candle, playing music.

Meditation & Mantra

I rejuvenate my mind & body.

Flowetry Prompts

How does sacred bathing benefit me?
How do I rejuvenate myself?

July 6th

Gentle movement

Engage in gentle movement like yoga, Thai chi, or dancing to honour and connect with your body. Focus on movements that make you feel connected, empowered and alive.

Meditation & Mantra

I appreciate my body.

Flowetry Prompts

What do I love & appreciate about my body?

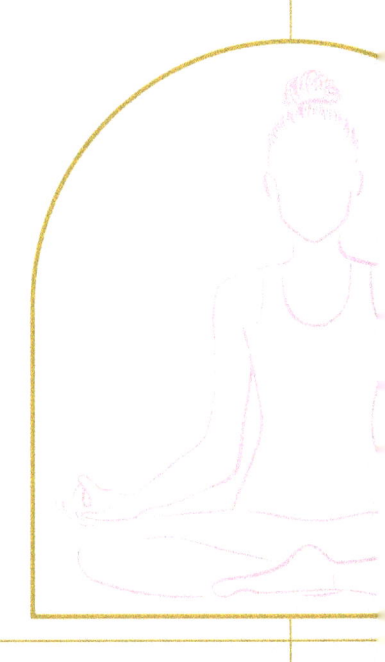

July 7th

Nourishing Activities

There are some experiences that nourish you and some that drain you.

Meditation & Mantra

I nourish myself wisely.

Flowetry Prompts

What nourishes me?
What depletes me?

July 8th

Release it

"Create a safe space to release any built-up emotions. Give yourself permission to journal, cry, scream into a pillow, or seek support from a trusted friend or therapist.

Meditation & Mantra

I release all that does not support my highest good.

Flowetry Prompts

What am I ready to let go of and why?

July 9th

Sisterhood connection

Find your tribe, spend time in meaningful connections with other women. Engage in supportive and empowering conversations.

Meditation & Mantra

I am connected.

Flowetry Prompts

Who is my tribe? What do I love about my tribe? What's my role in the tribe?

July 10th

Intuitive Practices

Your journaling practice gives your intuition a chance to show up, as we can't write as fast as we think, we have to slow down and this is a way to develop your intuition.

Meditation & Mantra

I am intuitive.

Flowetry Prompts

What would I like to say to my intuition? What do I love about my intuition?

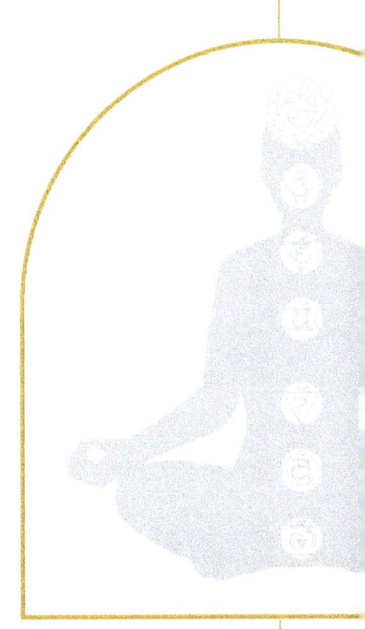

July 11th

Creative expression

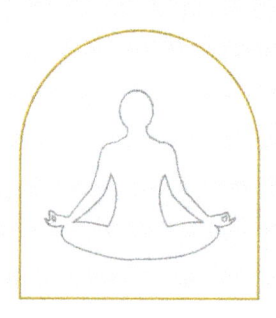

Choose creative outlets that feel good. Write, paint, dance, or engage in any form of artistic expression that allows you to tap into your feminine essence and explore your inner world.

Meditation & Mantra

I am creatively expressed.

Flowetry Prompts

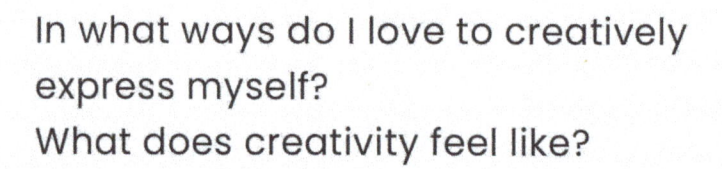

In what ways do I love to creatively express myself?
What does creativity feel like?

July 12th

Sacred Adornment

Today choose jewelry or clothing that makes you feel connected to the divine feminine. Choose symbols or crystals that represent the goddess energy.

Meditation & Mantra

I am in tune with my feminine energy.

Flowetry Prompts

How does it feel to step fully into my feminine energy?

July 13th

Silence

Having daily moments of silence is the biggest gift you can give yourself.

Meditation & Mantra

7 minutes of silence.

Flowetry Prompts

What do I love about being in silence?
What don't I like about being in silence?

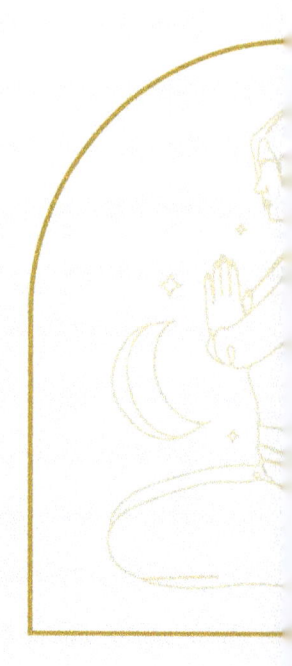

July 14th

Drop into your Heart

Out of your head and into your heart. Feel your way to peace, calm and love.

Meditation & Mantra

I am LOVE.

Flowetry Prompts

How does it feel to get out of my head and into my heart?

July 15th

OM

OM has several meanings. The sound of the universe, the sound of creation, the beginning of life, the sound of all sounds.

Meditation & Mantra

Using the in sound OM during your meditation. Sink with your breath and find a rhythm.

Flowetry Prompts

What are the universal laws I live my life by?

July 16th

Intent

Intent is the energy we carry through our day. I intend for things to go well.

Meditation & Mantra

My soul is filled with love, I am Love.

Flowetry Prompts

What are my intentions today?

July 17th

Soul Contribution

My Soul is deep and wholesome, I have so much to offer & contribute to all that my path crosses.

Meditation & Mantra

I embody my soul today.

Flowetry Prompts

What does my soul want to contribute to the world?
Who can I support?

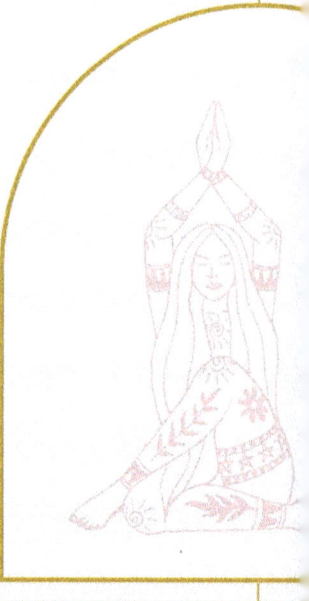

July 18th

Full Belly Breath

Connect to your breath, use your breath to cleanse you and uplift you.

Meditation & Mantra

I breathe with ease, I am safe and secure.

Flowetry Prompts

When do I feel most connected to myself?

July 19th

Heart's Prayer

Your heart knows what you need, your heart will guide and protect you. May you listen, may you follow your heart, May your heart be filled with love, courage and joy.

Meditation & Mantra

My heart is full with love, courage & joy.

Flowetry Prompts

What is my heart full of? What does my heart want me to know?

July 20th

Graceful Presence

Being present and allowing yourself to be soothed and held in the arms of Mother earth. Take your shoes off or lay on the earth. Be held, be soft, be gentle.

Meditation & Mantra

I am Graceful & Present.

Flowetry Prompts

Free write – Graceful Presence.

July 21st

Buddhi

Buddhi- inner wisdom & intellect. It's time to unlearn what you have been told and tap into your inner well of knowledge and wisdom. Resist the urge to second guess yourself.

Meditation & Mantra

I am...

Flowetry Prompts

Writing about a time when I listened to my inner wisdom. How did it make me feel?

July 22nd

Kriya

Kriya — effortless flow. Can you allow yourself to be in flow? No need to force or push, choose ease & flow.

Meditation & Mantra

I am in flow.

Flowetry Prompts

What am I resisting? Where in life do I need to let go and flow?

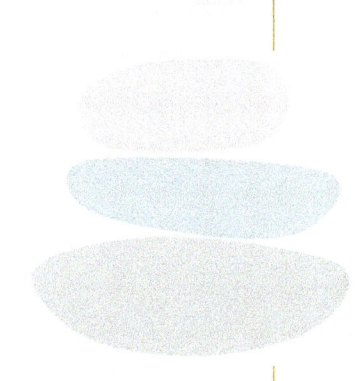

July 23rd

Buddha

Buddha – The one who is aware.

Meditation & Mantra

I am Aware.

Flowetry Prompts

What in my life needs my attention? What am I aware of?

July 24th

Daily Prayer

Dear Universe, use my hands, heart and words to bring peace to the others & the world. When I start to take things personal, please help me get out of my own way. Namaste.

Meditation & Mantra

Use my hands, heart, and words to bring peace today.

Flowetry Prompts

How could I bring peace and healing to my day?

July 25th

Soul Calling

Get quiet, listen, take notes and follow the crumbs. Your soul is always calling you.

Meditation & Mantra

I'm listing.

Flowetry Prompts

My soul knows my path. Free writing about my soul's whispers.

July 26th

Bless the world

Move your attention of yourself and shift it to blessing the world, sending love to all the other people & animals that we share mother earth with. Bless the oceans, plants, trees and wilderness with love.

Meditation & Mantra

I send loving kindness to the world.

Flowetry Prompts

Writing a blessing to the world, dedicating my morning pages to mother earth.

July 27th

Love of a Son

The love of your child leaves an imprint on your heart and soul, a love like no other. For me, the birth of my son encapsulates this. Happy Birthday, Sonny.

Meditation & Mantra

Love and connection.

Flowetry Prompts

Reflecting on the profound imprint a child's love has on your heart and soul.

July 28th

Find Yourself

STOP. Close your eyes and ask yourself: when I'm not busy or not productive, who am I?

Meditation & Mantra

Who Am I?

Flowetry Prompts

Who am I when I'm not busy?

July 29th

Inner Light

Connect to your inner light. Your inner light is free from hurt, sorrow and suffering. Welcome your inner light to sit with you in stillness.

Meditation & Mantra

I am light.

Flowetry Prompts

What does my inner light want me to know? Drawing my inner light.

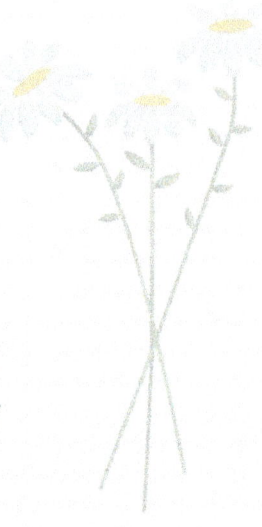

July 30th

Crack open

Your imperfections, cracks and scars, the seen and unseen hurts. These are your gifts. You are flawed and so am I.

Meditation & Mantra

I am...

Flowetry Prompts

How have my imperfections been a gift to me? In what ways have I turned a negative into a positive?

July 31st

Teacher

We have people in our lives that are our greatest teachers, even if it doesn't appear at first.

Meditation & Mantra

I am a student of life.

Flowetry Prompts

Who & what has been my greatest teacher?

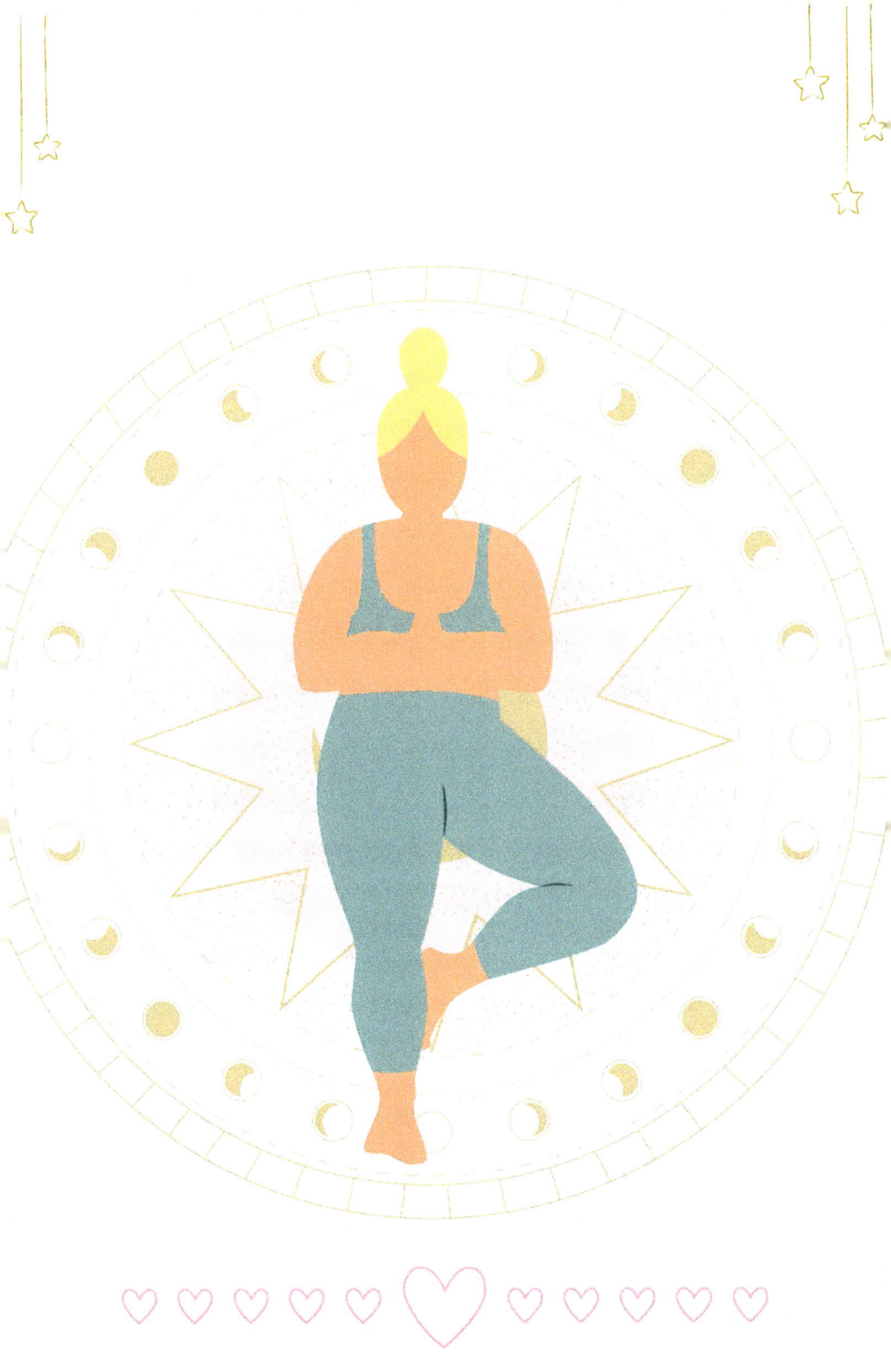

August

Holistic Wellness

Welcome to the sacred realm of 21 minutes of magic where our focus is on holistic wellness in the month of August. Where self-care dances hand in hand with mindful living. Embrace the morning sun as it kisses your skin, and feel the whispers of nature's secrets awakening your soul. Your daily ritual is a tender conversation with your being, a nurturing touch that feeds your spirit. With intuition as your guide and wisdom as your compass, commit to this journey of self-discovery. Embrace the power of consistency, for it unlocks your voice of. As you show up for yourself each morning, allow the gentle alchemy of time to weave magic, empowering you to blossom into the next version of yourself. Radiate sister! For the world awaits your luminous light.

August 1st

Go within

Harmony within= Balance throughout.
Seek internal harmony and it will flow into all areas of your life.

Meditation & Mantra

It's safe to go within.

Flowetry Prompts

Where in life do I need more harmony & balance?

August 2nd

Understanding Yourself

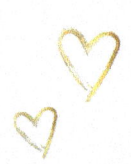

Understanding yourself and acknowledging your own worth is treating yourself with care & self love.

Meditation & Mantra

I am worthy of self love.

Flowetry Prompts

What do I understand about myself? Where do I fulfill my own needs?

August 3rd

Temple

You are a temple, embody your temple like a queen. Adore your temple.

Meditation & Mantra

I am a temple of love.

Flowetry Prompts

Writing a letter to my temple to tell her all the things I love about her and how grateful I am.

August 4th

Expectations

Let's replace expectations with intentions.

Meditation & Mantra

My intentions are wholesome & supportive.

Flowetry Prompts

I am listing all the expectations I have for myself and then rephrasing them as loving intentions.

August 5th

Let go of "Busy"

I do not fill my day with Busy. I am mindful of where I focus my energy & intentions.

Meditation & Mantra

My mind and body is spacious & light.

Flowetry Prompts

What does being busy feel like? What does spacious and light feel like?

August 6th

Illusion of time

We find ourselves in a hurry, under pressure and chasing the clock. Get curious about your relationship with time.

Meditation & Mantra

I have time & space.

Flowetry Prompts

What is my relationship with time? Is my mindset one of scarcity or abundance?

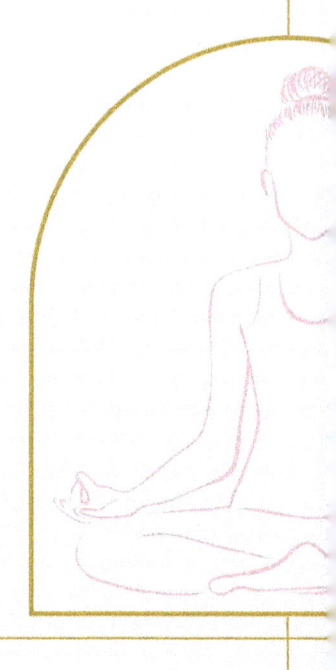

August 7th

Robust

I own my strength and I am unwavering. I have what it takes to choose a path less traveled. It's not easy, however it comes with ease.

Meditation & Mantra

I am Robust.

Flowetry Prompts

If I owned my strength and I was unwavering what would I do? What would I create?

August 8th

Vigour

Move with vigour today and ignite your passion for your life. Celebrate the spring in your step.

Meditation & Mantra

Today I move with vigour.

Flowetry Prompts

What in my life deserves my vigour, passion and joy?

August 9th

Nourish your mind

Open your mind to new and exciting people, places and experiences. Be open and let go of judgment. Be Curious.

Meditation & Mantra

I nourish my mind, body & soul.

Flowetry Prompts

Making a list of how I can nourish my mind.
What would I like to learn or explore?

August 10th

Make it happen

As I sit here writing this, I remind myself. Only YOU can make it happen. So write the book, do the thing!! You are the author of your life.

Meditation & Mantra

I am the author of my life.

Flowetry Prompts

Doing the thing - What's the thing I keep thinking about or talking about?

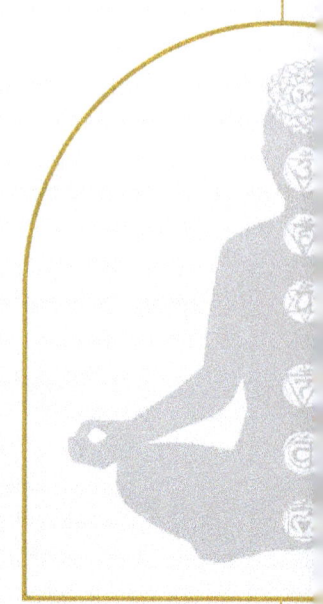

August 11th

Ten out of Ten

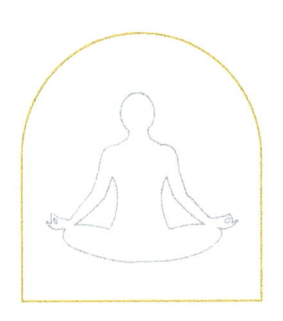

Today I will go for a 10/10 experience. A meal, an interaction, a hot shower, a smile, a belly laugh.

Meditation & Mantra

I create ten out of ten experiences in my life.

Flowetry Prompts

Writing down as many 10/10 experiences I have had or I would love to have.

August 12th

Beam of Light

Beam your light on all that crosses your path today. Shine your light on another, lift them up and acknowledge them for all that they bring to the world.

Meditation & Mantra

I am a beautiful beam of light.

Flowetry Prompts

Where and who will I beam my light upon today?

August 13th

Friendship

When we are in the presence of a true friend, they light you up, their company is like warm sunshine on your soul. Laughter, tears and everything in between are shared.

Meditation & Mantra

I am surrounded by love & support.

Flowetry Prompts

I am writing a letter of appreciation to all the friends, both past and present, in my life.

August 14th

The romantic

Today be romantic, lose the inner critic and see life through rose coloured glasses. Notice beauty wherever you go. Be soft.

Meditation & Mantra

I see beauty everywhere.

Flowetry Prompts

What and where do I see, feel, and experience beauty?

August 15th

Knock Knock

I believe we have all heard a gentle knock, a calling. Sometimes we answer and sometimes we don't. Listen deeply and tune into your inner knock.

Meditation & Mantra

I'm listening with my heart and soul.

Flowetry Prompts

Have I ever answered the call?
Have I ignored the call?

August 16th

Leave space

Block out the calendar, create space to do nothing or engage in activities you enjoy—read a book, sit, write, draw, and sleep.

Meditation & Mantra

I am spacious.

Flowetry Prompts

If I blocked out my calendar for a day, then a week, then a month, then a year, what would I do?

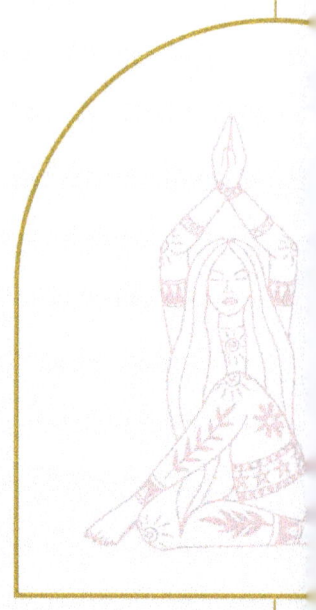

August 17th

Feather your nest

Make your nest beautiful, comfortable, cosy, light and filled with love.

Meditation & Mantra

My nest supports my life.

Flowetry Prompts

How do I feel about my nest? Where does my nest need attention?

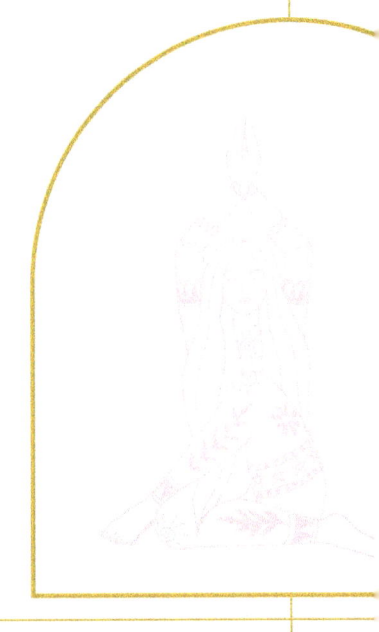

August 18th

Sunlight

Sunlight is medicine for the soul.
Seek it, bathe in it, enjoy it, admire it.

Meditation & Mantra

Sunlight lifts my energy.

Flowetry Prompts

What's my favorite season and why?

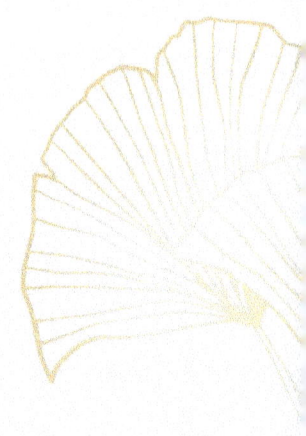

August 19th

Push Yourself

When was the last time you said Yes to something that scared you or pushed you outside your comfort zone. If not now? when?

Meditation & Mantra

Its safe for me to expand.

Flowetry Prompts

What's outside my comfort zone that I want to achieve, create or experience?

August 20th

Allies

Having allies that have your back and hold space for you. Is one of the greatest blessing you can have in your life.

Meditation & Mantra

Blessed with supportive allies, I thrive.

Flowetry Prompts

Who are my allies?
How do I support myself?

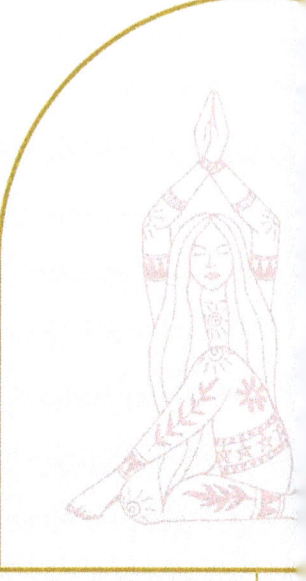

August 21st

Oracle

Over the years I have loved seeing clairvoyants, tarot readers, palm readers, anyone with a psychic ability. But to be honest I am the oracle.

Meditation & Mantra

I know what I know.

Flowetry Prompts

I trust myself because?

August 22nd

Wellness

Each of us is unique, requiring different elements to maintain wellness, health, and flow. Raising self-awareness about your wellness needs is an act of self-support.

Meditation & Mantra

I self support daily.

Flowetry Prompts

What supports my wellness? Daily practices? Weekly? Monthly & yearly?

August 23rd

Devotional Practice

Commend yourself for your devotion to 21 Minutes of Morning Magic practice. Movement, stillness & reflection. You have created a wonderful start to the day.

Meditation & Mantra

I am devoted to myself and my wellbeing.

Flowetry Prompts

What do I love about my morning practice? What am I devoted to?

August 24th

Slow YOU

Hurry up and slow down! When we are so used to running at a pace it can be hard to slow down. Your nervous system need you to slow down.

Meditation & Mantra

It's safe for me to slow down.

Flowetry Prompts

In what ways can I slow down in my life? What area of life needs me to create space?

August 25th

Flow YOU

Being in flow is where the answers come and the path unfolds before you. There are no efforts required.

Meditation & Mantra

I am in flow.

Flowetry Prompts

What does being in flow feel like? Where do I flow? Who do I flow with?

August 26th

Grow You

You are the one to tend to your own garden. Plant seeds, place them in the sun, water them, feed them, and enjoy the fruits of your labor.

Meditation & Mantra

I tend to my inner garden.

Flowetry Prompts

What seeds have I planted? How am I taking care of my garden?

August 27th

Fertile

You are full of bountiful ideas and creativity. You are ripe and full of ideas and ready to bring them to life.

Meditation & Mantra

I am bountiful.

Flowetry Prompts

What creative ideas would I like to bring out into the world? What does creativity feel like?

August 28th

Invitation

We are constantly being invited to grow and expand. It's your time to accept the invite from the universe and bless the world with your presence.

Meditation & Mantra

I am here and ready to shine.

Flowetry Prompts

What and where in life am I holding back? How can I express myself and my creativity today?

August 29th

Change

Love, loss, life & lesions happen. Some are painful and some are exquisite. We must feel all the emotions to know the difference.

Meditation & Mantra

I feel.

Flowetry Prompts

What have I loved and lost?
Where has life been exquisite?

August 30th

Unbound

It's time to free yourself from old ties and stories. Step forward with ease & grace.

Meditation & Mantra

My heart & soul is free.

Flowetry Prompts

What old ties and stories am I ready to let go of? Where do I feel most free?

August 31st

Admiration

Life has many beautiful people, places and experiences that we get to admire, adore and applaud. Open your heart and mind to adore this wonderful life you have.

Meditation & Mantra

I admire, adore & applaud my life.

Flowetry Prompts

What do I admire, adore & applaud in my life?

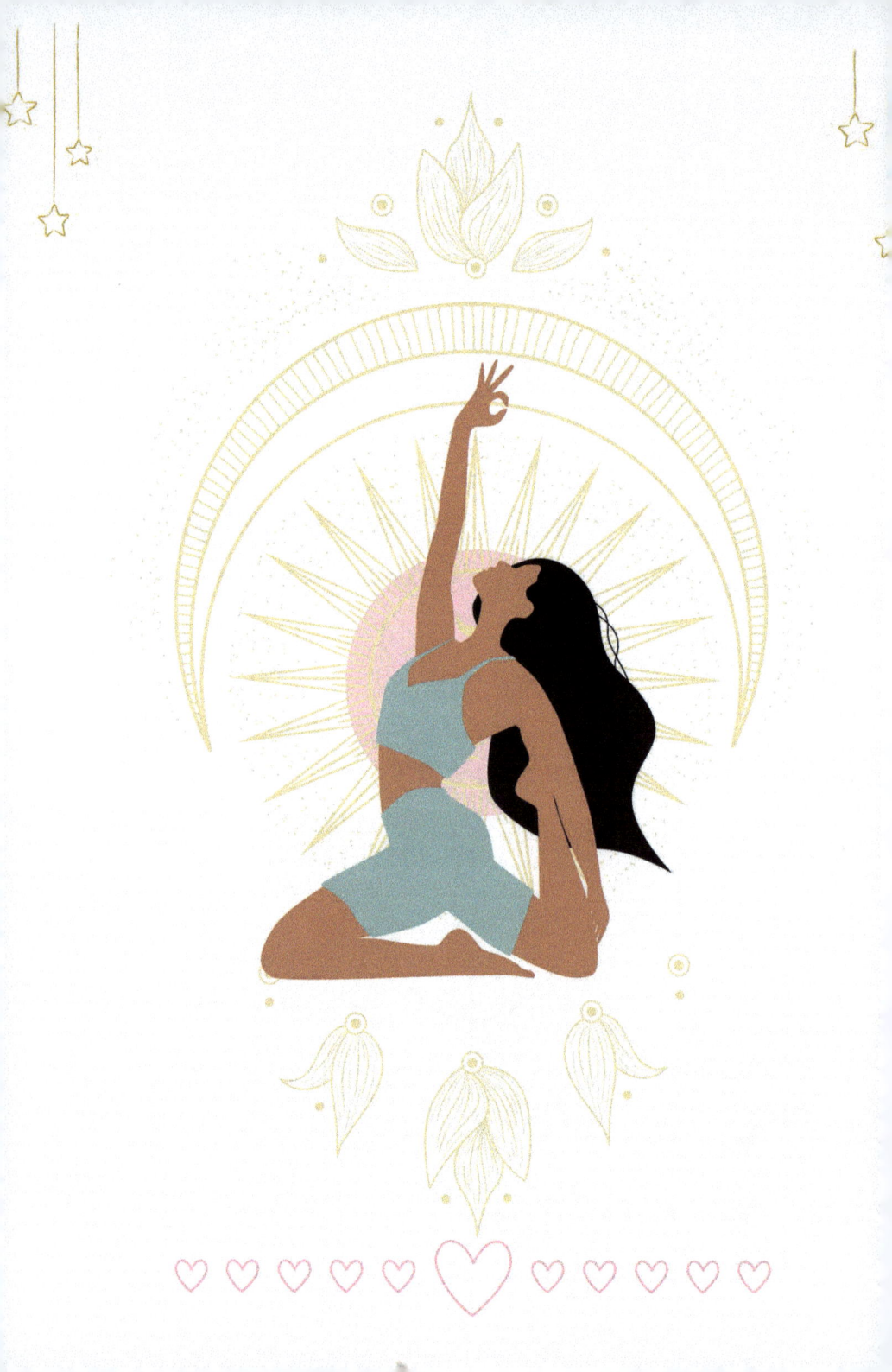

September

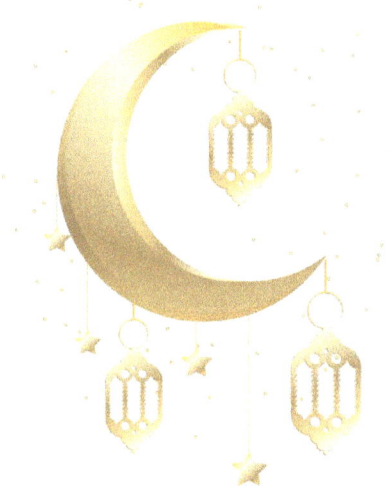

Home & Living Space

Your home is more than just walls and a roof; it is a profound extension of your being. Within its embrace, the very essence of your soul finds solace and expression. The arrangement of each corner, the choice of colors, and the cherished mementos tell a story that echoes your unique journey. As you create a sanctuary of warmth and belonging, remember that your dwelling breathes with your spirit. Just as a tree extends its roots into the earth, your home delves into the depths of your identity, a sacred space where your heart and soul truly reside.

September 1st

Spring Clean

My Nana Ursula had a yearly ritual that the house was to be decluttered and cleaned from head to toe to welcome spring.

Meditation & Mantra

I embrace growth and renewal.

Flowetry Prompts

How can I harness this energy of spring to bring about positive changes and growth in my life?

September 2nd

Home

Identity and Self-Expression. Your home often reflects our identity and personality through its design, decor, and arrangement, we express our taste, values, and individuality.

Meditation & Mantra

I am home.

Flowetry Prompts

What do I love about my home?

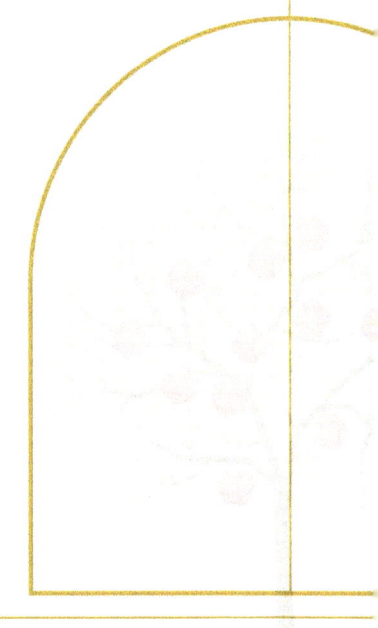

September 3rd

North

The North star has been a symbol of guidance and direction for seekers and travelers finding their way home.

Meditation & Mantra

I know my north star.

Flowetry Prompts

Where & who do I feel most at home?

September 4th

East

The East is associated with new beginnings, renewal, enlightenment, and spiritual awakening.

Meditation & Mantra

I welcome new beginnings with an open heart.

Flowetry Prompts

I visualize myself stepping into a new beginning with confidence and courage, describing the person I see.

September 5th

South

In a spiritual sense, the south direction is often associated with the element of fire, passion, transformation, and personal growth. As you look to the south ask yourself what am I passionate about?

Meditation & Mantra

I embrace the fire within me and ignite my soul's purpose.

Flowetry Prompts

Writing to the fire in my belly and asking her what and how she wants to show up in the world.

September 6th

West

In the west direction we can associate with the element of water, emotions, introspection, reflection and letting go.

Meditation & Mantra

I surrender to the natural flow of life.

Flowetry Prompts

What emotions am I holding onto, and why? Both positive and negative emotions?

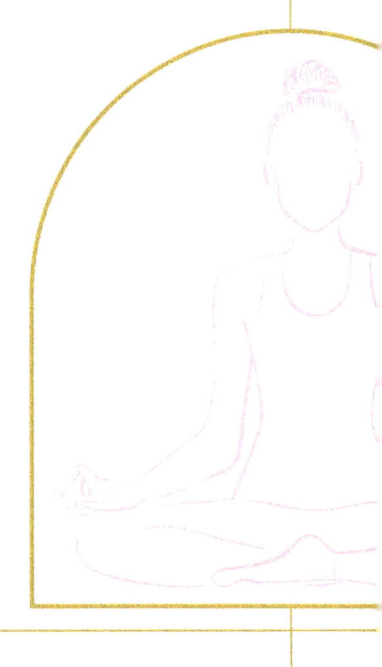

September 7th

Room with a view

The power of visualization. What's your perfect room with a view.

Meditation & Mantra

Bring your attention to your third eye " Imagine your room with a view".

Flowetry Prompts

Drawing and writing about my room with a view. Rolling around in appreciation & gratitude.

September 8th

Intuitive Space

Creating a sacred space to nurture your spiritual practice, reflect and allow your intuition to whisper into your ear.

Meditation & Mantra

The quieter, I get the more I hear.

Flowetry Prompts

What does my ideal sacred space look like, feel like, and smell like? What do I need to support my intuition?

September 9th

Evoke Creativity

Your spiritual home can be filled with beautiful art, literature, or objects that inspire you and evoke creativity and personal growth.

Meditation & Mantra

My spiritual home inspires creativity and growth.

Flowetry Prompts

What inspires creativity and personal growth in my spiritual home?

September 10th

Haven

Our home is our haven. A place of profound inner connection, a positive atmosphere where we recharge our energy, feel grounded and have fun & connection.

Meditation & Mantra

My home is my haven.

Flowetry Prompts

What does my home haven feel like? If I could make any changes what would they be?

September 11th

Secluded Garden

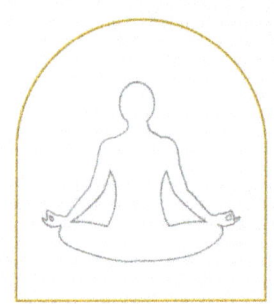

Finding a little patch of garden is quiet and peaceful. Sit and admire the grace & harmony of mother nature.

Meditation & Mantra

Nature's grace, balance and harmony in this space.

Flowetry Prompts

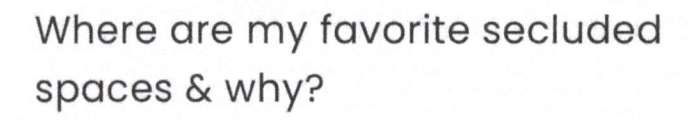

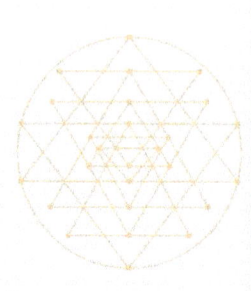

Where are my favorite secluded spaces & why?

September 12th

Harbor

A harbor is a safe and secure place that offers comfort and stability in our lives. It holds a deeper meaning as a refuge, a source of love, and connection—where we recharge and rediscover our true selves.

Meditation & Mantra

Our home anchors our soul.

Flowetry Prompts

What significance does my home hold for you?

September 13th

Protection

Similar to a snail that carries its home on its back, providing the ability to retreat at any time, your home offers a safe place to withdraw from the world.

Meditation & Mantra

It's healthy for me to retreat.

Flowetry Prompts

How does it feel to retreat from the outside world? How does my soul respond?

September 14th

Refuge

Spiritual refuge, a sacred place, within my home, my soul finds comfort and time to restore.

Meditation & Mantra

I am home.

Flowetry Prompts

Writing about the feelings that reinforce the spiritual essence of my home and how it nourishes my inner being.

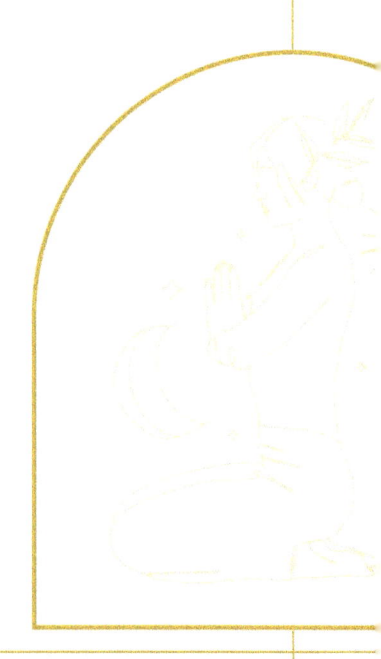

September 15th

Home Rituals

There is a sense of peace and contentment in the mundane tasks that keep our home life in flow. Enjoy the humdrum.

Meditation & Mantra

Home is my sanctuary.

Flowetry Prompts

How do these rituals contribute to my overall sense of well-being and belonging?

September 16th

Light & Dark

Each area of my home has lightness and darkness. A beautiful balance of action and stillness.

Meditation & Mantra

I am Luminous.

Flowetry Prompts

How does my home luminate my soul?

September 17th

Extension of You

Your home is an extension of you. Be bold, be proud and enjoy creating a space you love. You are worth it.

Meditation & Mantra

I love where I live.

Flowetry Prompts

What does my home say about me? What changes or adjustments could I make?

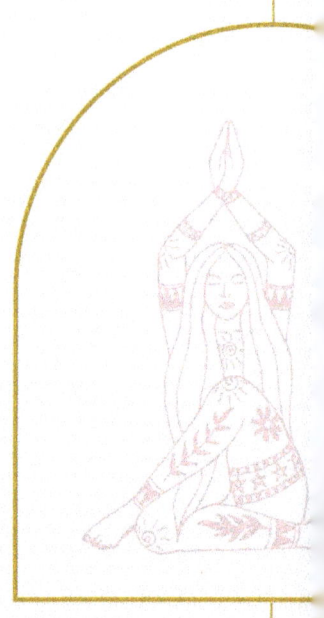

September 18th

Nana Ursula

Your favorite childhood memories may have been experienced in your grandparents home, aunties or friends. I know for me this was the case. In particular my Nana Ursula, a small house but full of LOVE.

Meditation & Mantra

I am filled with love.

Flowetry Prompts

Writing about my grandparents/ family's home that brings back sweet memories.

September 19th

Ideal Home

An ideal home can mean many different things to many different people. It could be about functionality, a look, a feel or a lifelong project.

Meditation & Mantra

I am worthy of my ideal home.

Flowetry Prompts

Writing about my ideal home, its location, attributes, and how it makes me feel while supporting me.

September 20th

Favourite Room

My favourite room in my home is a sacred space, where my soul finds inspiration, ideas and a space where I create and I am filled with joy.

Meditation & Mantra

I am an inspired creator.

Flowetry Prompts

When I'm in my favourite room in my home I...

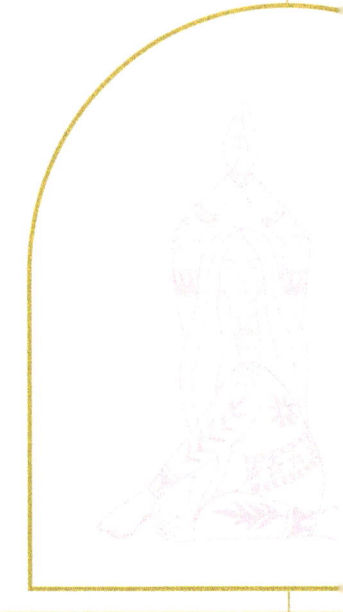

September 21st

Castle

It may not be big, it may not be trimmed with gold and the finest of fabrics but it's mine. It's my castle.

Meditation & Mantra

Sacred castle, fortress of my soul.

Flowetry Prompts

Writing about my castle.

September 22nd

It feels like Home

Ahhhh... It feels like home, it smells like home. I know I'm home.

Meditation & Mantra

I am home.

Flowetry Prompts

What does coming home feel, smell & look like to me?

September 23rd

Dream Bedroom

In our dream bedroom's embrace, hearts intertwined as the world fades finding solace in love's restful sanctuary.

Meditation & Mantra

I love my bedroom.

Flowetry Prompts

Describing and drawing in detail my dream bedroom.

September 24th

Water is energy

I cherish those moments when beneath the shower's gentle cascade, inspiration flows and my soul softly shares its beautiful ideas.

Meditation & Mantra

I am open to new inspiration and ideas.

Flowetry Prompts

Dedicating my morning flowetry to water. How is water a gift in my life?

September 25th

Soulful Kitchen

Our kitchens are the heart and soul of the home. Family gathers and hearts meet. Long morning cuddles happen while waiting for the kettle to boil.

Meditation & Mantra

I love our kitchen's heart and soul.

Flowetry Prompts

Writing about my memories, moments and magic of my family in the kitchen.

September 26th

Creative Study

A space that is created just for you. Ideas come and work is done.

Meditation & Mantra

I am making progress.

Flowetry Prompts

What's my dream study/creative space? What does it look and feel like?

September 27th

Cosy living room

In the cosy living room, a feeling of comfort and connection. A sanctuary for cherished moments, introspection & relaxation.

Meditation & Mantra

I am centered and connected.

Flowetry Prompts

How do the walls of my home inspire my dreams and nurture my growth?

September 28th

Grand Entry

Keep the entryway clutter-free for positive energy flow to flow into your home.

Meditation & Mantra

I feel the energy flow with ease.

Flowetry Prompts

What should my perfect front door and entryway look and feel like?

September 29th

Exquisite outdoors

Place vibrant plants at the patio's entrance to invite positive energy and beauty.

Meditation & Mantra

I love growth in my life.

Flowetry Prompts

What do I know to be true when I spend time outdoors?

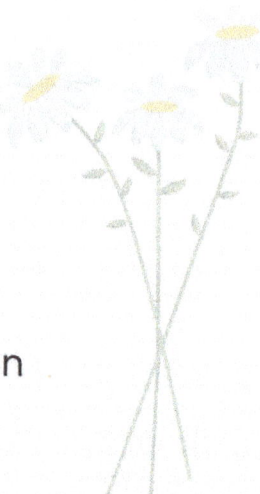

September 30th

Extension of YOU

Your home is deeply connected to you and who you are. It's an extension of your personality and essence.

Meditation & Mantra

I appreciate all that I am and all that I have.

Flowetry Prompts

If my home had a voice what would it want me to know?

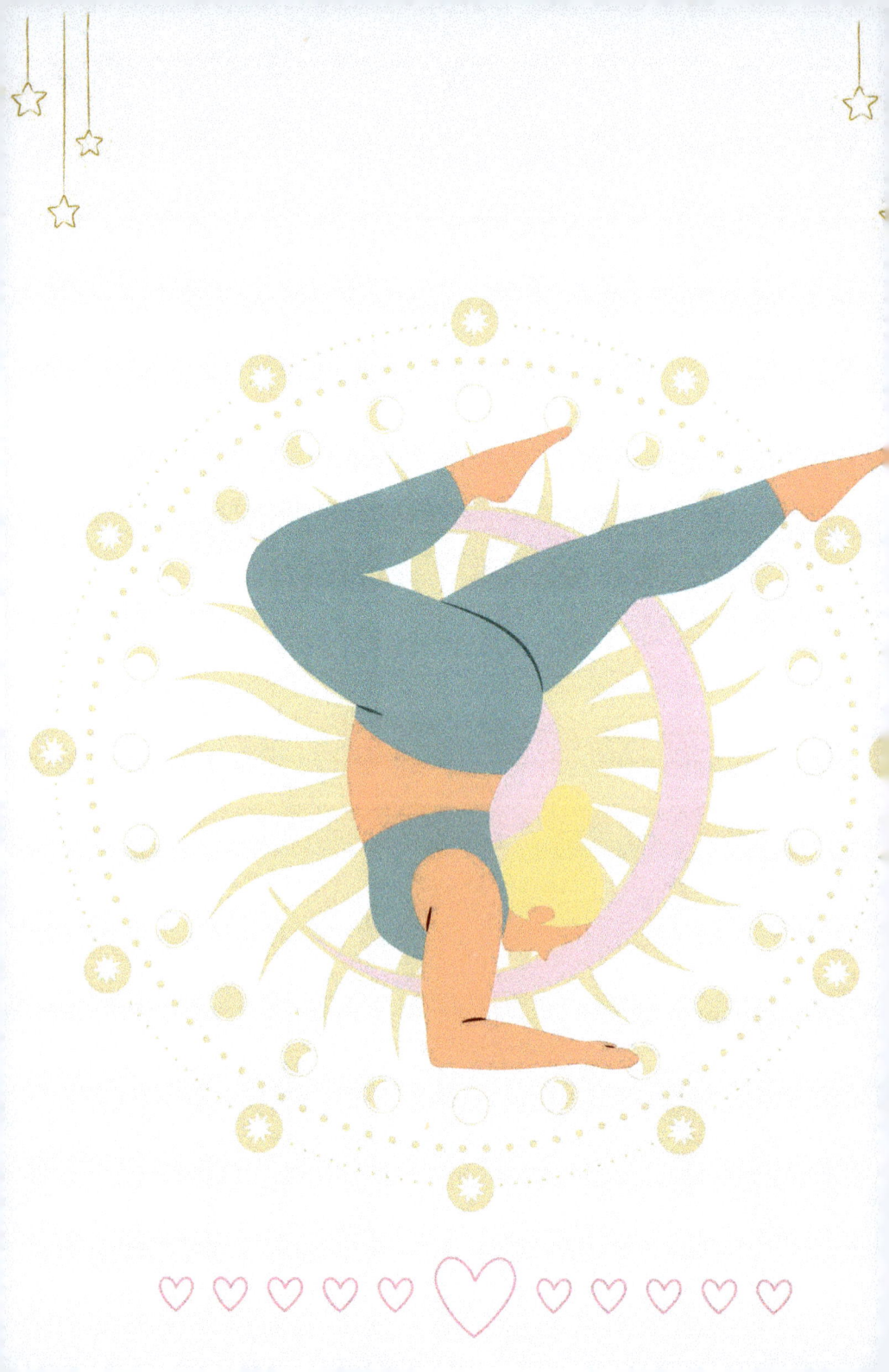

October

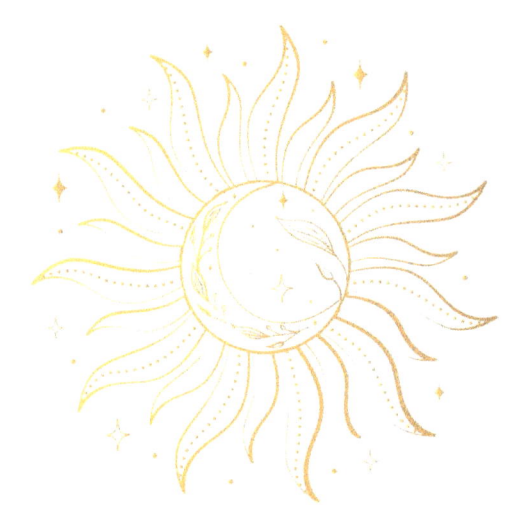

Relationships & love

Just as the sun rises in the morning sky, love and connection illuminate the dawn of our daily routines. In the gentle rituals of waking, we discover the profound beauty of human bonds. Love is the tender embrace shared with a partner as we rise from slumber, a reminder that our hearts are forever entwined. Connection is the whispered greetings to family and friends, a harmonious symphony of voices that echo in our souls. As we embark on the journey of a new day, let us carry the warmth of love and the strength of connection with us, infusing our morning rituals with the soulful essence of human connection.

October 1st

Love

May you do all things with love, compassion & joy firstly to yourself and then to others.

Meditation & Mantra

I am LOVE.

Flowetry Prompts

Writing about LOVE.

October 2nd

Romantic Date

I believe Romantic Dates are of great value to the bond & connection between two lovers. Keep the sweetness "Sweet".

Meditation & Mantra

Love & connection.

Flowetry Prompts

Writing a list of sweet romantic dates I would love to experience.

October 3rd

Sacred Union

When you meet your match and come together there is a sacred connection between you both. Cherish these moments as they will last a lifetime in your heart and soul.

Meditation & Mantra

I cherish this moment.

Flowetry Prompts

What does Sacred Union mean to me?

October 4th

Location of Love

There are many cities & places that exude love and romance. Is it cinque Terre in Italy, Edinburgh in Scotland or the Gold Coast Australia? What is it for you?

Meditation & Mantra

Love is everywhere.

Flowetry Prompts

What are the most romantic places I've been or would love to visit?

October 5th

First Love

I believe our first love is one of the most exciting experiences ever. The pounding heart, you can't eat, you can't sleep and you can't get enough of each other.

Meditation & Mantra

I am love.

Flowetry Prompts

What do I remember about the first time I fell in love ?

October 6th

Be First

Be the first one to show love, warmth & affection. Express how you feel.

Meditation & Mantra

It's safe to express my feelings.

Flowetry Prompts

How do I feel in my relationships? Are there any tweaks I could make and why?

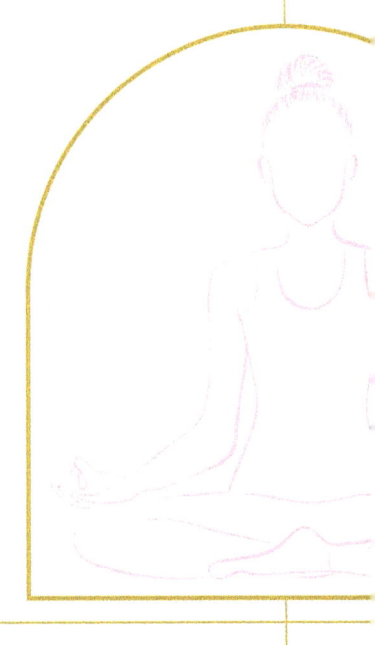

October 7th

Compromise

One might say that this is the key to a happy marriage.

Meditation & Mantra

I am open.

Flowetry Prompts

What are the elements of a wonderful relationship with myself and others?

October 8th

Spontaneous

Spontaneity rekindles the excitement of discovery and keeps the flame of passion burning bright, reminding us that love is a dynamic, ever-evolving journey.

Meditation & Mantra

I embrace spontaneity.

Flowetry Prompts

What does spontaneity in my relationships look and feel like?

October 9th

Embrace

Amidst life's ups and downs, our love story deepens with devotion and resilience. Embrace the good, the bad & the ugly.

Meditation & Mantra

I embrace all experiences.

Flowetry Prompts

What valuable lessons have I gained from the good, the bad, and the ugly moments in life?

October 10th

Personal Growth

We have the most personal growth when we are in a relationship with another. We learn so much about ourselves.

Meditation & Mantra

I am growing.

Flowetry Prompts

Taking time to reflect on how far I have come.

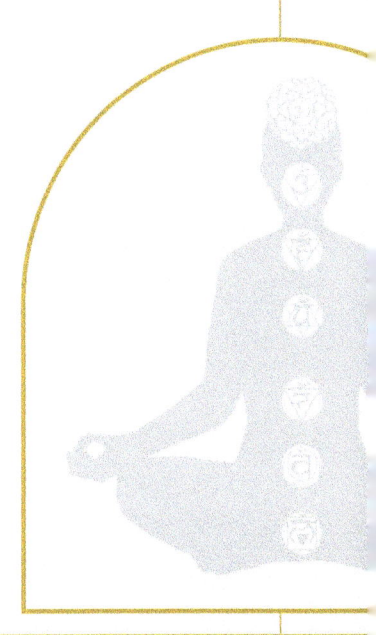

October 11th

Values

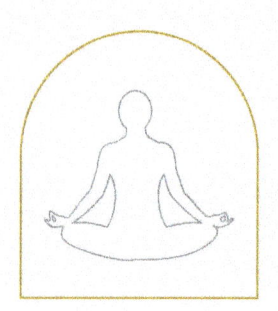

In a soulful relationship that thrives on connection, shared values are the compass guiding our journey.

Meditation & Mantra

I value soulful connection.

Flowetry Prompts

What do I value in a partner and why?

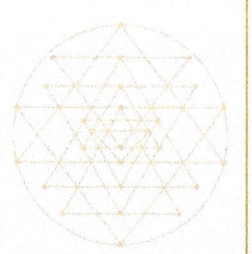

October 12th

Circle of Love

I often describe myself as half a circle, with my significant other completing the other half. We're a match, fitting together despite being opposites.

Meditation & Mantra

Opposites complete circles.

Flowetry Prompts

How do my differences bring balance to my relationship?

October 13th

Unspoken

A deep connection doesn't always need words. It's a look, it's a tilt of the head, it's a smirk.

Meditation & Mantra

I am in tune.

Flowetry Prompts

Reflecting on the soulful connections I have in my life.

October 14th

Prince Charming

You are your own Prince Charming. You are strong, smart and thriving.

Meditation & Mantra

I am thriving.

Flowetry Prompts

Writing my fairytale, a tale of a thriver and a go getter.

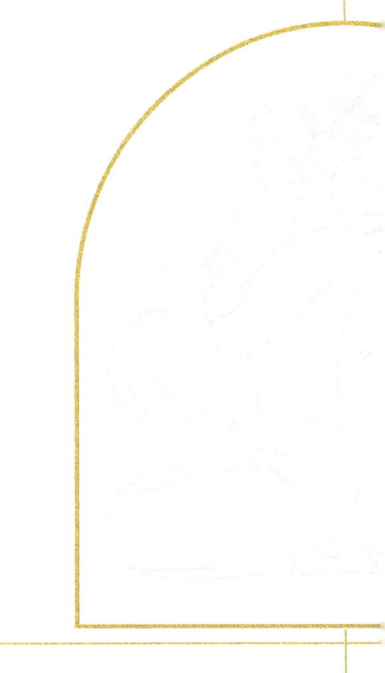

October 15th

Be Held

Allow others to support you physically, emotionally, or spiritually. It's healthy for you to receive support.

Meditation & Mantra

I am supported.

Flowetry Prompts

What can I do to deeply replenish today? How can I accept support in my life?

October 16th

Words Of Love

Talk to yourself as if you were your significant other. Words of respect, kindness, care & love.

Meditation & Mantra

I feel love emit from my heart.

Flowetry Prompts

Writing all the things I love about myself. What makes me unique?

October 17th

Don't hold back

Hold nothing back from the people you love. Take time to tell your parents all the things they got right.

Meditation & Mantra

Gratitude and forgiveness.

Flowetry Prompts

Focus on all the things your parents got right. What are some of the positive things your parents taught you?

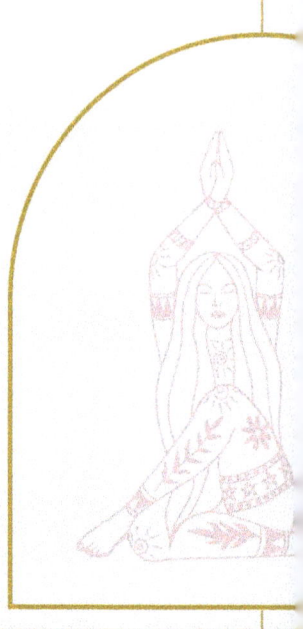

October 18th

Grandparent

A grandparent is like a parent, but with an extra dose of leniency and a heart full of joy. They're always ready to indulge and spoil you, taking the time to nurture and create lasting memories.

Meditation & Mantra

Love, Joy, Cherish.

Flowetry Prompts

Writing about my grandparents, a grandparent figure in my life, or the kind of grandparent I want to be.

October 19th

I choose YOU

Choose a life partner whose qualities and values resonate with the deepest essence of your soul, creating a harmonious and spiritual connection for a lifetime of shared purpose and love.

Meditation & Mantra

I am harmonious.

Flowetry Prompts

What do I love and adore about my life partner or future life partner?

October 20th

Soft landing

On those days when it all feels too much, we all need a soft landing and a loving hug or ear to hold us.

Meditation & Mantra

Love surrounds me.

Flowetry Prompts

Writing about a moment when I found comfort in the support of others and what it taught me about the importance of connection and compassion.

October 21st

Magnetic

Certain people, places, and spaces hold a special place in our hearts, drawing us closer with a gentle, loving pull. In return, our very presence exudes warmth and affection.

Meditation & Mantra

I am magnetic.

Flowetry Prompts

What people, places and spaces am I drawn to and why?

October 22nd

Shared Dreams

Consider the pride you take in your accomplishments with a loved one. Celebrate the shared dreams you have fulfilled together and reflect on how they have strengthened your bond

Meditation & Mantra

I am a powerful creator.

Flowetry Prompts

What dreams do I have?
What dreams do I have with my significant other?

October 23rd

Deep Dive

Dive into the depths of your heart and feelings. How can you become more connected to your own emotions and heart space, mirroring the depth of a spiritual person in touch with their inner self?

Meditation & Mantra

My heart is open.

Flowetry Prompts

Diving deep into my heart, what does my heart want and need and why?

October 24th

Burn Brightly

Feeling of being in a relationship where the love burns brightly, making you and your partner feel like there's no one else in the world.

Meditation & Mantra

I feel...

Flowetry Prompts

How can I nurture passion in my life?

October 25th

Admiration

Admiration is the radiant sunbeam that warms the garden of our hearts, nurturing the blossoms of love and respect.

Meditation & Mantra

Strength, Love, Resilience.

Flowetry Prompts

Thinking about someone I deeply admire. How has this admiration influenced my life and relationships positively?

October 26th

Butterflies in your Belly

Butterflies in your belly: Sweet anticipation, Magic in motion, Love's delightful dance.

Meditation & Mantra

I am joyfully expressed.

Flowetry Prompts

Writing about the sweetness of a first date, first kiss and the excitement.

October 27th

Charisma

Charisma is the radiant magnetism that lights up hearts and inspires souls.

Meditation & Mantra

I am radiant.

Flowetry Prompts

Recalling a charismatic moment in my life and reflecting on the impact it had on me.

October 28th

Loyalty

Soulful loyalty, the unwavering commitment that comes from the depths of the heart, has the power to enrich and deepen one's life.

Meditation & Mantra

I am unwavering in my commitment to self.

Flowetry Prompts

Where in life am I loyal and unwavering?

October 29th

Gentleness

Gentleness is the tender touch that nurtures the roots of a soulful relationship, allowing love to bloom and trust to flourish.

Meditation & Mantra

I allow myself to be nurtured.

Flowetry Prompts

Reflecting on the role of gentleness in a soulful relationship. How does it impact connections?

October 30th

Companionship

Companionship, love, and care form the foundation of a beautiful and enduring connection.

Meditation & Mantra

My foundation is strong.

Flowetry Prompts

What I appreciate most about the companions and companionship in my life is..

October 31st

Divine appointment

The universe weaves its plan, guiding us to a divine appointment with someone special. There are no coincidences!

Meditation & Mantra

I radiate love.

Flowetry Prompts

Writing about my "Someone Special" and all the things I love about them.

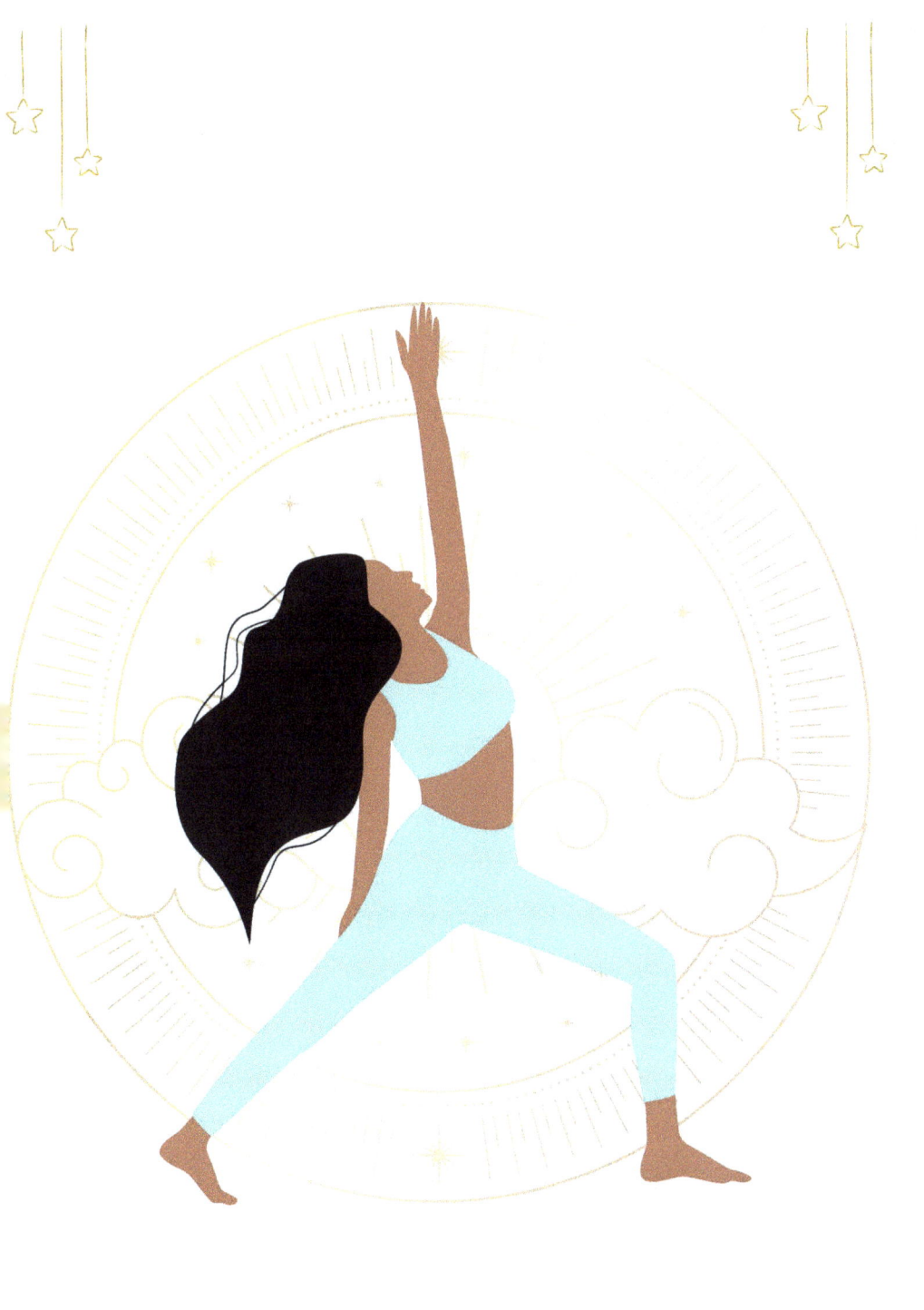

November

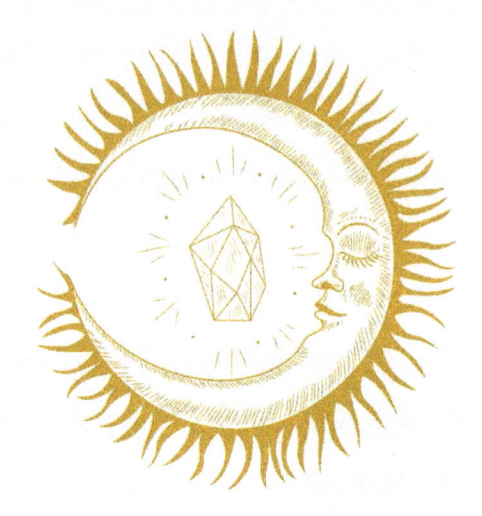

You're worth it

Your self-worth and self-acceptance are at the core of your being, deeply rooted in the profound truth that your very existence makes you a divine goddess. Embrace this profound wisdom that you are inherently enough, just as you are. As you dance through life, allowing your passions to bloom and your spirit to soar, you become a beacon of authenticity and joyful contribution to the world. Unburden yourself from doubt and bask in the safety of being your true self. In your unique radiance lies your strength, your beauty, and your limitless worth as a goddess, spreading happiness and joy to all you touch.

November 1st

Replenish

Rest, recoup, replenish and treat yourself like you would your beloved.

Meditation & Mantra

I am worthy of rest.

Flowetry Prompts

In what ways can I rest, my energy, spirit and soul?

November 2nd

Congregation

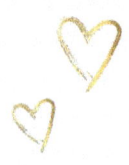

When you soar with eagles, you will become an eagle. It is said that Eagle spirit animal is the power of the Great Spirit; the connection to the Divine.

Meditation & Mantra

I am an Eagle.

Flowetry Prompts

What's my spirit animal?

November 3rd

Self Respect

Self-respect is recognizing your inherent worth from a spiritual perspective, embracing the divine within you.

Meditation & Mantra

I am worthy & divine.

Flowetry Prompts

How can I strengthen my self-respect and connection to self?

November 4th

Precious Self

Be gentle and kind with your precious self, you are doing your best and it's more than good enough.

Meditation & Mantra

Love and Kindness.

Flowetry Prompts

Letting my words flow about all the wonderful things I'm doing and how amazing I am.

November 5th

Right

You have been right, you have been wrong, but you have grown and evolved and you are right on track.

Meditation & Mantra

I am right on track.

Flowetry Prompts

What am I sure about in my life?

November 6th

Transition & Expansion

I am in a constant state of transition because I value personal growth and I love to expand my mind and heart.

Meditation & Mantra

I am open to change.

Flowetry Prompts

What if I accepted where I am at right now?

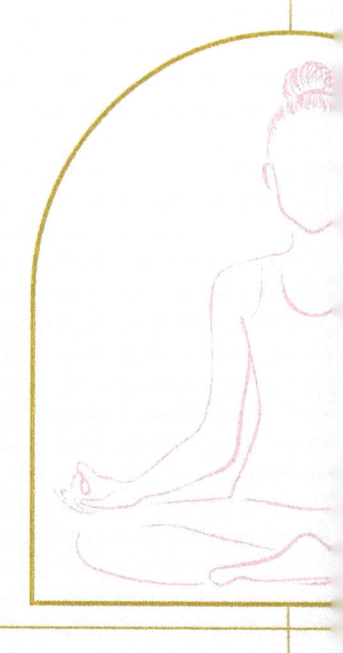

November 7th

It's Done

What is done is done. It's over and I choose to move forward with a smile on my face and love in my heart.

Meditation & Mantra

I am moving forward.

Flowetry Prompts

What if I decided to write a new story, what would it say?

November 8th

Fabulous Future

Set your eyes on the horizon, your future is bright and waiting for you. Go for it!

Meditation & Mantra

I am excited about my future.

Flowetry Prompts

What's in my heart? What do I want my future to look & feel like?

November 9th

Trust in Self

Deep within myself I have all the answers. When I get quiet and I tune in, I hear the whispers of my Voice of Wisdom.

Meditation & Mantra

I trust myself.

Flowetry Prompts

Dig deep. What do I know to be true?

November 10th

Self-reflection

Self-reflection involves delving deeply into your inner self to discern your true value and purpose.

Meditation & Mantra

I embrace inner wisdom.

Flowetry Prompts

If I were to stop measuring my worth or success in relation to others, how would my life look & feel?

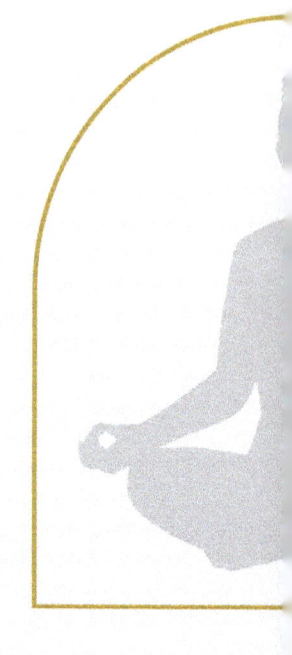

November 11th

Decisions

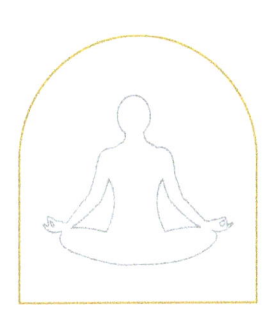

Sometimes it's hard to decide. What can I do? What do I want to do? Decision fatigue is real!

Meditation & Mantra

I connect with my soul's essence.

Flowetry Prompts

What if I had 3 choices? What are they and why?

November 12th

Keep it light

Easy breezy, light and easy...Laugh at yourself often, lean into joy.

Meditation & Mantra

I am easy breezy, light and easy

Flowetry Prompts

Where in my life could I lighten up and why?

November 13th

Fearless

Fear has given me feedback on what's important to me. Fear has lovingly shown me the path to my heart's desires.

Meditation & Mantra

I am fearless.

Flowetry Prompts

Reflecting on the ways fear has illuminated my soul's true desires and jotting down what I've learned.

November 14th

Wild Flower

Blossom, unapologetically, as your own wild flower, dancing to the rhythm of your soul's unique song.

Meditation & Mantra

I blossom no matter where I'm planted.

Flowetry Prompts

Where am I blossoming in life and why?

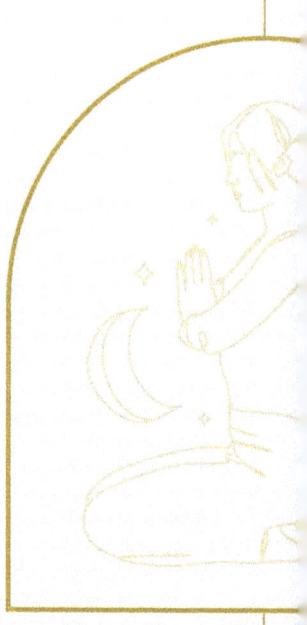

November 15th

Unearthed

We will be unearthed at some time in our life. I trust that in these moments of adversity, the true me will stand up and be counted.

Meditation & Mantra

I count.

Flowetry Prompts

Reflecting on a time when I was unearthed and how I grew from this.

November 16th

Guide

Be your own guide. You have an inner captain of your ship that can navigate the seas. Tune in and course correct or adjust your sails when needed.

Meditation & Mantra

I listen to my inner guide.

Flowetry Prompts

What does my inner guide want me to know? Do I need to course correct or adjust my sails in my life at the moment and why?

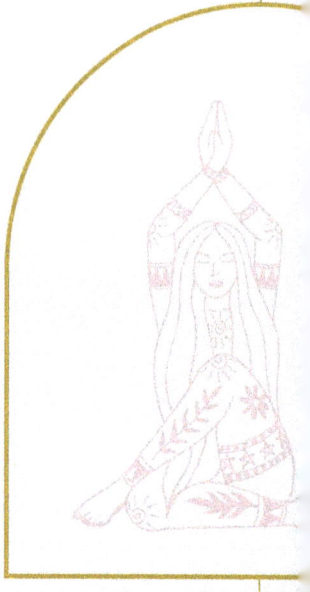

November 17th

Radiate

Illuminate the world with your brilliance. It eagerly awaits your radiant light, yearning for you to bring forth your extraordinary gifts and shine brightly.

Meditation & Mantra

I radiate love out into the world.

Flowetry Prompts

What am I radiating out into the world?

November 18th

Advocate

Be your own advocate. Champion yourself. Be as supportive to yourself as you are to others.

Meditation & Mantra

I embrace my Inner Strength.

Flowetry Prompts

Where in your life could I advocate or champion myself more & why?

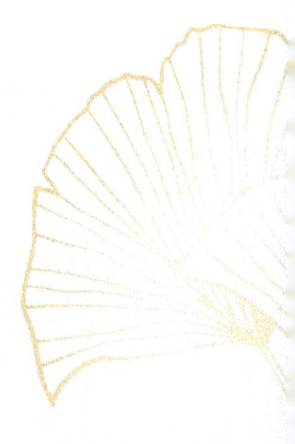

November 19th

Pioneer

Embrace your inner pioneer, with a passion for creating what has not been done before, forging new pathways in the spirit of divine creation.

Meditation & Mantra

I am a Pioneer with Passion.

Flowetry Prompts

Tapping into my creativity. What inspires innovation and trailblazing in my life and why?

November 20th

Hedonist

A hedonistic soulful goddess is someone who passionately embraces life's pleasures while exuding a spiritual and graceful presence.

Meditation & Mantra

I embrace my inner Hedonist.

Flowetry Prompts

Reflecting on my blend of pleasure and spirituality. How do they intertwine in my life?

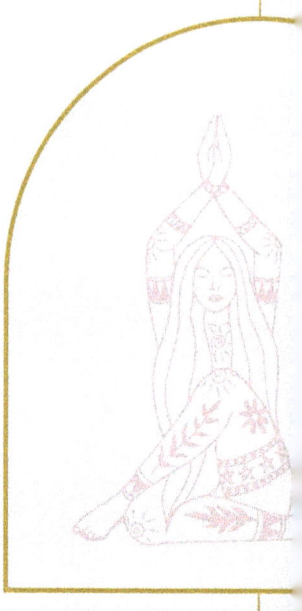

November 21st

Inner Artist

Bring forth your inner artist, express yourself in all that you do. Celebrate your creativity.

Meditation & Mantra

I welcome my inner artist to express herself.

Flowetry Prompts

Embracing my inner artist. What inspires my creativity at this moment? What have I always wanted to try and why?

November 22nd

Companion

Companionship, a cherished gift that enriches the soul.

Meditation & Mantra

I cherish all that I am and all that I have.

Flowetry Prompts

What are the qualities of a wonderful companion?

November 23rd

Visionary

Hold a beautiful vision for your future. Take time to envision how you want things to unfold.

Meditation & Mantra

I envision a beautiful future.

Flowetry Prompts

What's my vision? What would I like to see unfold in my life?

November 24th

Daughter

My beautiful daughter, you are the sweetest and most angelic soul I know. Your gentle presence, your peaceful creative energy, and your cheeky giggle make my heart sing. Dedicated to my Ruby, with all my love.

Meditation & Mantra

Love & Joy.

Flowetry Prompts

Reflecting on having a daughter or being a daughter. What does it mean to me?

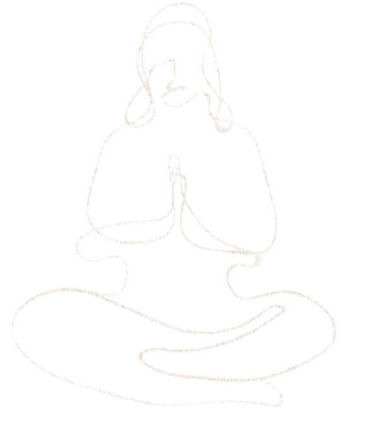

November 25th

Mystic

The modern-day mystic, with unwavering intuition as their guide, uncovers profound spiritual truths in a rapidly changing world.

Meditation & Mantra

My intuition is unwavering.

Flowetry Prompts

What does your intuition want me to know?
What mystic experiences have I had or heard of?

November 26th

Rebel Heart

With a rebel heart, I reject conformity and wholeheartedly embrace the untamed spirit within, cherishing the freedom to be unapologetically me.

Meditation & Mantra

I embrace who I am.

Flowetry Prompts

Where does my rebel heart come out and why? What does my rebel heart need?

November 27th

Challenge

Challenges are sent to help us grow and expand into the next version of ourselves. Not always comfortable however worth it.

Meditation & Mantra

I rise & shine.

Flowetry Prompts

What area of life do I want growth in?

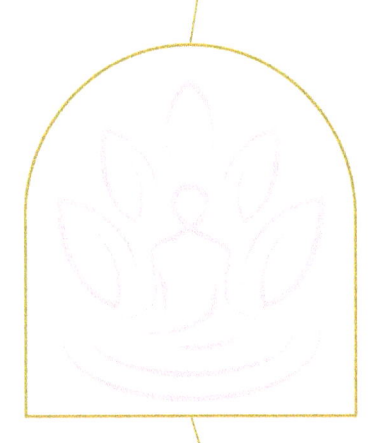

November 28th

Day Ahead

Think about your day ahead. It's your day. What will you do? Where will you go? Whose life will you touch?

Meditation & Mantra

I am love.

Flowetry Prompts

It's my day. What will I do? Where will I go? Whose life will I touch?

November 29th

I Promise

Make a declaration to yourself, what promise do you hold yourself to?

Meditation & Mantra

I put myself first.

Flowetry Prompts

How will I treat myself and take care of my mind, body & soul?

November 30th

Written in the stars

There are some things in life that are written in the stars. For me it is my beloved husband. I cherish, love & adore this soul with all that I am. Happy Birthday Brendon.

Meditation & Mantra

I cherish us.

Flowetry Prompts

What was written in the stars for you? Who do you love, adore & cherish and why?

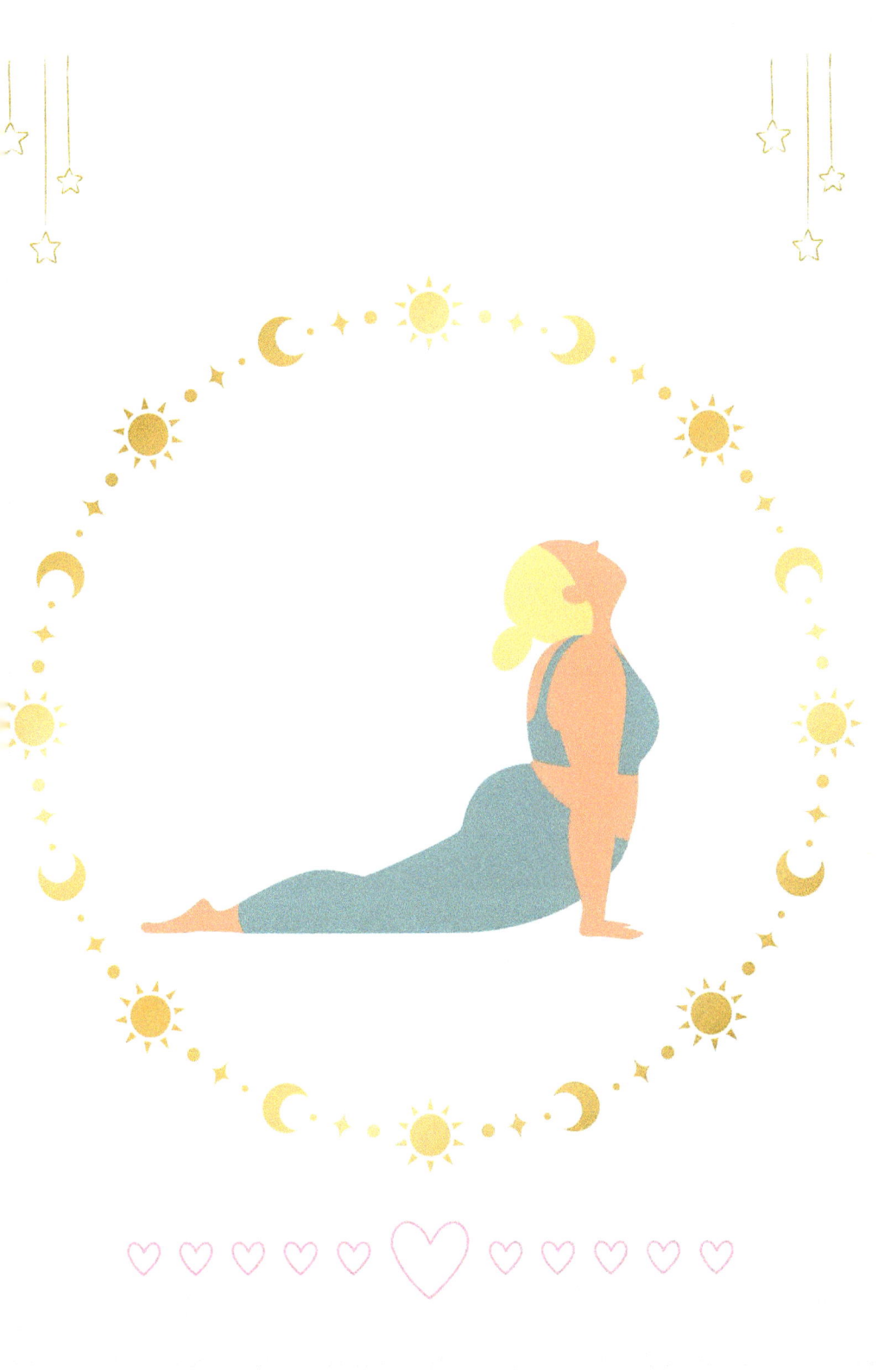

December

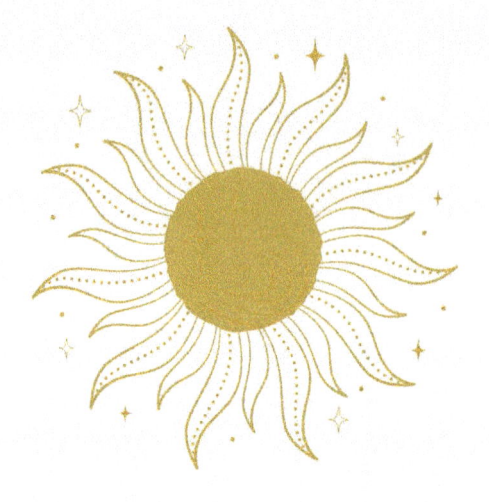

Powerful presence

We, as women, stand tall with a powerful presence that radiates happiness, joy, and soulfulness. Our hearts are tender, yet our strength is unshakable, like the steadfast roots of a mighty tree. We make a difference in the lives of our friends, family, and the world itself, sometimes in the most unassuming ways. Our collective spirit is a force to be reckoned with, reminding the world that our resilience and kindness are catalysts for positive change, shaping a better future for all.

December 1st

Day of Birth

Birthdays are the day that we celebrate ourselves and our loved ones. For all the mothers out there, a day we remember oh to well..
The day we gave birth.

Meditation & Mantra

I am a miracle.

Flowetry Prompts

How do I feel about Birthdays? What's my favorite Birthday memory?

December 2nd

No More

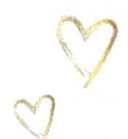

EXCUSES... We all from time to time make up excuses.

Meditation & Mantra

Inspired action feel great.

Flowetry Prompts

What excuses do I want to release? What's holding me back?

December 3rd

Know Yourself

When you know yourself really well you stop saying yes to things that you don't like.

Meditation & Mantra

I am self-aware.

Flowetry Prompts

Why do I say yes when I should say no?

December 4th

Sound Decisions

Wisdom comes from experience and self-reflection. A powerful woman uses her wisdom to make sound decisions and guide others with a sense of purpose.

Meditation & Mantra

I lead with wisdom.

Flowetry Prompts

Reflecting on how wisdom shows up in my life and what that means to me.

December 5th

Cultivate your powerful presence

Curiosity is a powerful tool for self-discovery. Stay curious about your powerful presence in the world.

Meditation & Mantra

I am powerful.

Flowetry Prompts

How can I cultivate my powerful presence? Where would I like to be more present in my life?

December 6th

Confident Body Language

Stand in your power, be present and exude confidence in this gorgeous body that you are in.

Meditation & Mantra

I am present.

Flowetry Prompts

What makes me feel confident and why?

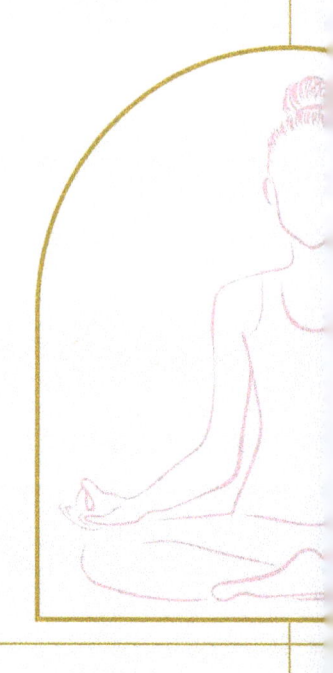

December 7th

Real Work

It's easy to be displeased and judge yourself. The real work is to Love where you're at.

Meditation & Mantra

I accept and I appreciate myself.

Flowetry Prompts

What do I need to accept about myself? How can I practice more self acceptance?

December 8th

Body Buddhaful

Wise words of Buddha. Your body is precious. It is your vehicle for awakening. Treat it with care.

Meditation & Mantra

I am Buddhaful.

Flowetry Prompts

Writing about how buddhaful my body, mind and spirit is. Expressing love to myself.

December 9th

Say it Daily

Say this to yourself often: I am a divine being, worthy of love and acceptance, just as I am.

Meditation & Mantra

I am enough just as I am.

Flowetry Prompts

Making a list of things I can say to myself daily.

December 10th

Sacred Vessel

My body is a sacred vessel, and I honour and appreciate it in all its uniqueness. I listen to its need and nourish accordingly.

Meditation & Mantra

My body is a sacred vessel.

Flowetry Prompts

Taking the time to honour my sacred body vessel, writing down all the things I love and respect about my sacred body.

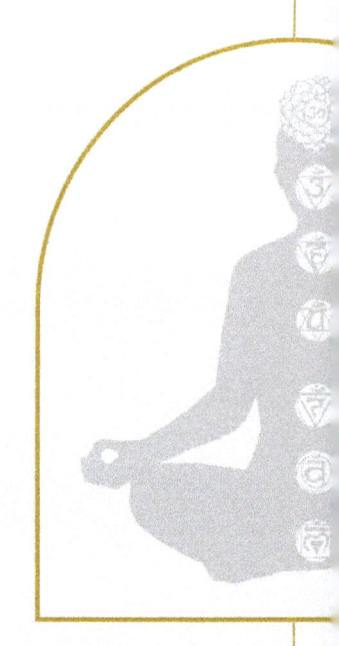

December 11th

Radiate Beauty

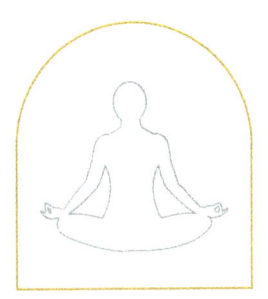

I radiate inner beauty and self-confidence, which shines brighter than any external standard.

Meditation & Mantra

Today I shine bright.

Flowetry Prompts

When you shine bright how does that look & feel?

December 12th

Release

I release all judgment and criticism of my body, embracing every part with love and appreciation.

Meditation & Mantra

I release all that holds me back.

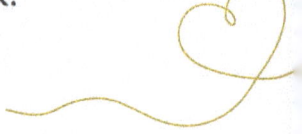

Flowetry Prompts

What do I need to release in order to flourish?

December 13th

Determined

Every day, I grow stronger in self-love, knowing that my worth is not determined by my appearance.

Meditation & Mantra

I am growing stronger.

Flowetry Prompts

How have I grown stronger in my life? What supports my growth?

December 14th

Reservoir of Love

I am a reservoir of love, kindness, and compassion, and I direct this energy first towards myself.

Meditation & Mantra

I am a reservoir of love.

Flowetry Prompts

With the power of words on a page. Filling my own reservoir with love.

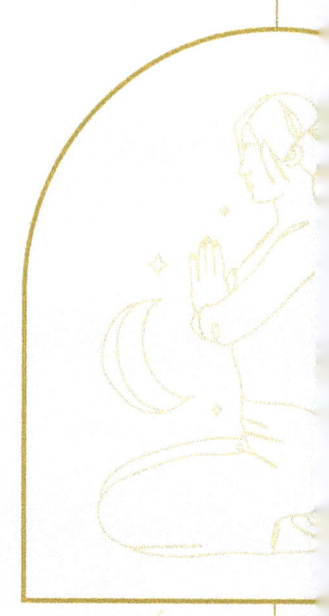

December 15th

Past

I forgive myself for any past self-criticism and embrace the journey of self-love and self-acceptance.

Meditation & Mantra

I embrace the journey of self acceptance.

Flowetry Prompts

Writing a letter to myself and forgiving myself for past criticism and judgment.

December 16th

Spiritually Enriched

My spiritual journey is enriched by my love for myself as I learn to love and appreciate all parts of my being.

Meditation & Mantra

I am spiritually enriched.

Flowetry Prompts

When I live a spiritually rich life how does it look & feel?

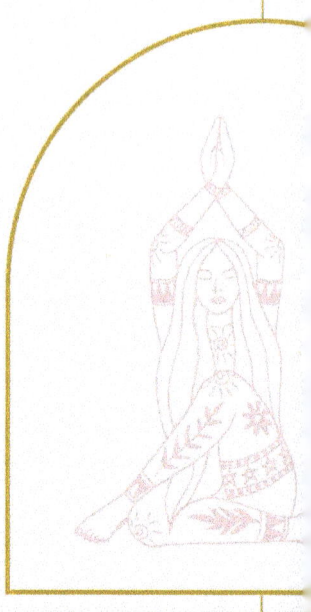

December 17th

Utmost Love

Today, I vow to respect and treat myself with the utmost love and care, as I am all that and a bag of chips.

Meditation & Mantra

I treat myself with respect.

Flowetry Prompts

Making a vow to myself & my body.

December 18th

Reflection Powerful presence

Your presence is powerful, keep your eye on your hopes & dreams. The new year approaches and you have what it takes.

Meditation & Mantra

I am a powerhouse.

Flowetry Prompts

Reflecting on the past year. Identifying moments when I felt empowered. Setting intentions for the upcoming year, outlining how I'll continue to embrace my power.

December 19th

Reflection: You're worth it

It's your birthright to be seen and take up space. You are enough because you were born.

Meditation & Mantra

I am more than enough.

Flowetry Prompts

Reflecting on the past year: How did I honour my worthiness, and where did I fall short?

December 20th

Reflection: Relationships & love

In my opinion there is no greater gift than to have heartfelt soulful honest relationships that bring laughter, joy and connection.

Meditation & Mantra

I am love.

Flowetry Prompts

Reflecting on the past year: In what ways did I nurture my soulful connections, and where did I encounter challenges?

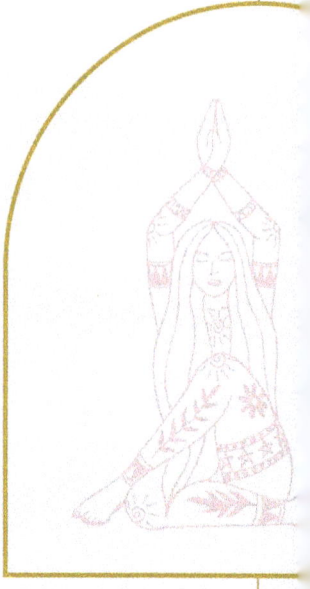

December 21st

Reflection: Home & living space

Living in a beautiful supportive home that is a haven from the outside world. Your safe place, your soft landing.

Meditation & Mantra

I am surrounded by beauty.

Flowetry Prompts

Reflecting on my past year at home. How has my living space been a comforting sanctuary?

December 22nd

Reflection: Holistic wellness

Our wellness is the big picture. Your wellness is equal parts body, mind & soul.

Meditation & Mantra

I am well, whole and content.

Flowetry Prompts

Reflecting on my wellness over the past year. Did I nurture my mind, body & soul?

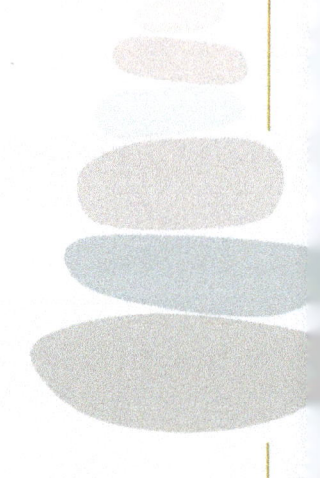

December 23rd

Reflection:
Money prosperity & abundance

We are in constant flow. Money, prosperity & abundance is circulating everywhere. The practice of appreciation has more abundance show up.

Meditation & Mantra

Embrace life's richness.

Flowetry Prompts

Reflecting on the past year: Where have I had money, prosperity & abundance show up in my life?

December 24th

Reflection: Spirituality & Daily practice

A daily spiritual practice is a chance for your voice of wisdom, your intuition to speak to you. You have your own answers. You know what's best for YOU.

Meditation & Mantra

I trust my voice of wisdom.

Flowetry Prompts

Reflecting on the past year: How have I cultivated my spirituality? How has my daily practices supported me?

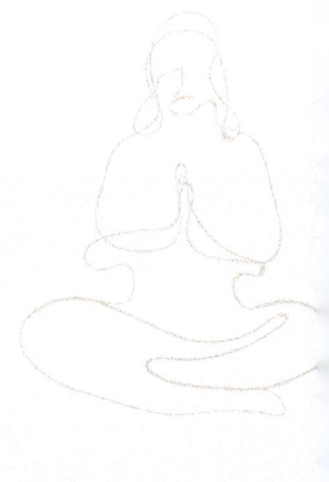

December 25th

Peace & Joy

May your day be filled with peace, love, connection and joy.

Meditation & Mantra

I am love, peace & joy.

Flowetry Prompts

How do I feel today? What do I most appreciate about my life?

December 26th

Reflection: Purpose & passion

Living a purposeful, passionate life is a sure way to never grow tired, old or bored. You were born to live a fully expressed life.

Meditation & Mantra

I am living a fully expressed life.

Flowetry Prompts

Reflecting on the past year: How did I express my purpose & passion in the past year?

December 27th

Reflection: Fun & play

The sound of laughter and the expression of joy and humour has the ability to heal and soothe the soul.

Meditation & Mantra

I am full of fun, joy & happiness.

Flowetry Prompts

Reflecting on the past year: What gave me the most fun, joy and pleasure this past year?

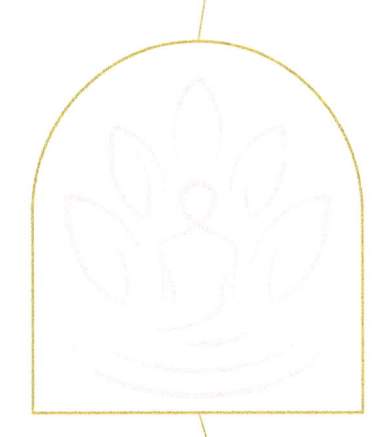

December 28th

Reflection: Self-love & Compassion

Compassion for oneself, a fundamental form of self-love, nurtures inner well-being and fosters a positive relationship with one's own being.

Meditation & Mantra

I embrace self-compassion daily.

Flowetry Prompts

Reflecting on the past year: What is one act of self-compassion I'm proud of?

December 29th

Reflection: Commitment to self

Keeping our word and staying the path isn't always easy. Stay true to your own word. Choose to be committed everyday.

Meditation & Mantra

I am true to my word.

Flowetry Prompts

Reflecting on the past year: Was I committed and consistent? What is my promise to myself this coming year?

December 30th

Reflect on heart's desire

Your dream, goals, passion and purpose are worth your attention and your time.

Meditation & Mantra

I honour my heart.

Flowetry Prompts

Reflecting on the past year:
Did I honour my dreams, goals and passion? What am I proud of?

December 31st

Reflect on the year that was

Today, make a decision to look back on this year with joy! Make a decision to speak of all the goodness this year brought to you.

Meditation & Mantra

I love the life I have created.

Flowetry Prompts

What have been my highlights of this year?

About the author:

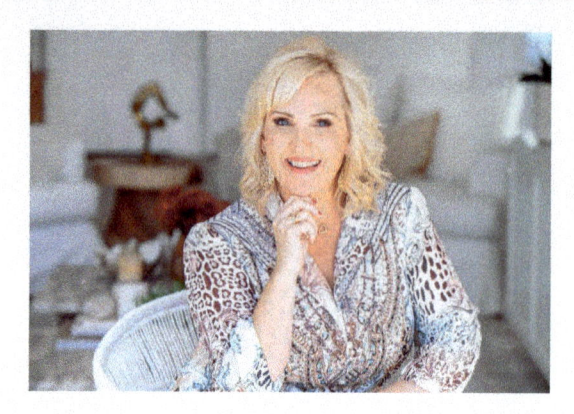

Emma Walkinshaw is a dedicated Transformational Coach, Accredited Yoga Instructor, and a dynamic entrepreneur with a passion for empowering women. As the Founder of the transformative "21 Minutes of Morning Magic" and "Embody Me Program," she creates spaces for growth and self-discovery. Emma also leads the "Body Love Revolution Online Summit" and hosts the inspiring "Wholehearted Retreat" for women here in Australia and Internationally.

With a decade of coaching experience backed by ICF certification, Emma's journey in personal development and business is marked by her entrepreneurial spirit, which ignited when she launched her first business at 23. As an Accredited 200hr Yoga Instructor, she has shared her expertise through over 1,000 hours of teaching, fostering a connection between mind, body, and spirit.

Emma's true passion is in guiding women to elevate their self-awareness and self-confidence, challenging toxic diet culture, and encouraging the acceptance of their authentic selves. She empowers her clients to break free from societal standards and pursue their heart's desires, regardless of size and shape. Her impact is profound, as she has inspired her students to embark on diverse journeys, including starting businesses, writing books, discovering their purpose, initiating new careers, and fostering deeper connections. Emma Walkinshaw's work is a testament to her commitment to fostering a world where women feel empowered, confident, and aligned with their true selves.

Where to find Emma?

✨Morning Magic Community
✨Embody Me Program
✨1:1 Coaching Sessions
✨Wholehearted Yoga & Wellness Retreats
✨Celebrate a Sister Podcast

Join Emma on a journey of self-discovery through her enriching retreats, workshops, and personalized 1:1 coaching. Be part of our community and explore the path to personal growth and connection. Visit her website and take the first step toward a soulful adventure with us!

🌐 https://www.emmawalkinshaw.com.au/home

📷 emma_walkinshaw

f Emma Walkinshaw Transformational Coach

🎙 Celebrate a Sister Podcast

▶ Emma Walkinshaw-Transformational Coach

For bulk book orders email:
teamwalkinshaw@gmail.com

Printed in Australia
Ingram Content Group Australia Pty Ltd
AUHW010951250624
396169AU00004B/5

9 780646 895239